Administration of Programs in Speech-Language Pathology and Audiology

Herbert J. Oyer, Editor
The Ohio State University

Prentice-Hall, Inc., Englewood Cliffs, New Jersey 07632

Library of Congress Cataloging-in-Publication Data

Administration of programs in speech-language pathology
    and audiology.

    Includes bibliographies.
    1. Speech, Disorders of—Patients—Services for—
Administration.   2. Hearing disorders—Patients—
Services for, Administration.   I. Oyer, Herbert J.
RC427.A36 1987   362.1'9685'5   86-16885
ISBN 0-13-006446-7

Editorial/production supervision and
    interior design: Marianne Peters
Cover design: 20/20 Services, Inc.
Manufacturing buyer: Harry P. Baisley

Printed in the United States of America

10 9 8 7 6 5 4 3 2 1

ISBN   0-13-006446-7   01

Prentice-Hall International (UK) Limited, *London*
Prentice-Hall of Australia Pty. Limited, *Sydney*
Prentice-Hall Canada Inc., *Toronto*
Prentice-Hall Hispanoamericana, S. A., *Mexico*
Prentice-Hall of India Private Limited, *New Delhi*
Prentice-Hall of Japan, Inc., *Tokyo*
Prentice-Hall of Southeast Asia Pte. Ltd., *Singapore*
Editora Prentice-Hall do Brasil, Ltda., *Rio de Janeiro*

Contents

Preface   vii

1   Administration: Some Initial Observations   1
     Herbert J. Oyer

2   The Development of Speech-Language Pathology
and Audiology in the United States   13
     John J. O'Neill

3   Some Reflections of Leadership   30
     D.C. Spriestersbach

4   Administration of Speech-Language-Hearing
Programs within the University Setting   36
     Edward J. Hardick
     Herbert J. Oyer

iii

5   Public School Speech-Language-Hearing Administration   54
     Gloria L. Engnoth

6   Community-Based Speech-Language-Hearing Clinic
     Administration   84
     Fred H. Bess

7   Administration of Community Hospital
     Speech-Language-Hearing Programs   100
     Twila Strandberg Griffith

8   Administration of a Military-Based Program of Speech-
     Language Pathology and Audiology   129
     Roy K. Sedge

9   The Veterans' Administration Program in Speech
     Pathology and Audiology   157
     Henry E. Spuehler

10   Research and Training Programs of the National
     Institute of Neurological and Communicative Disorders
     and Stroke   174
     Raymond R. Summers

11   American Speech-Language-Hearing Association
     and Its National Office   190
     Frederick T. Spahr

12   Summary Comments   205
     Herbert J. Oyer

     Appendix I   208

     Appendix II   210

Appendix III: Code of Ethics of the American Speech-Language-Hearing Association – 1983   212

Index   217

Preface

The purpose of this book is to make available a discussion of the topic of administration as it pertains to programs of speech-language and hearing. The book has been developed as a result of the need expressed by both professionals and students for a discussion of the principles and processes, as well as the special problems, that characterize the administration of programs in various settings. The settings discussed in this book include a university, a hospital, a public school, community-based clinics, military and veterans' centers, a government agency, and the national office of the American Speech-Language-Hearing Association. There may be those who believe that the chapters dealing with military and verterans' programs should have been combined. However, they deal with two quite different clientele and are administered under two different administrative systems.

In addition to the descriptions of administrative concerns in specialized settings, there are general discussions related to the topic of administration, such as leadership and a history of the development of the field of speech-language and hearing.

Those who have contributed to this book are experienced administrators and each a Speech-Language Pathologist and/or Audiologist. Their discussions flow naturally from their years of service as administrators. The topics they highlight and the concerns that they express are reinforced by their own experiences and observations. Also to be thanked are those who reviewed this book for their helpful comments: Elaine L. Brown-Grant of Northwestern University; Sophia Hadjian of the University of North Carolina at Chapel Hill; and Mary Jo Schill of the University of North Dakota.

The editor's hope is that the discussions in this book will be helpful to those who have assumed administrative responsibilities for speech-language and hearing programs in one of the settings described and to those persons to whom they report. It is further hoped that students in training will have a better understanding of the administrative framework within which they will work one day. For those who aspire to administrative posts, it is hoped that they will find this book to be beneficial in acquainting them with the concepts of administration and leadership required of those who direct speech-language-hearing programs in various settings.

Herbert J. Oyer

1 Administration: Some Initial Observations

Herbert J. Oyer*

Administration of organizations as a topic of formal study in programs of higher education is commonly undertaken within Education, Business, and Public Administration. Only recently has the need for formal discussion of administration in relation to programs of speech-language and hearing been given greater consideration.

The following chapters present discussions of the challenges and the problems of administration in relation to a variety of settings where education, service, and/or research in speech-language and hearing are the central concerns. But first let us consider several topics briefly, all of which are germane to the discussion of administration of speech-language and hearing programs.

ASSUMPTIONS RELATED TO ADMINISTRATIVE STRATEGY

Like most organizations, the speech-language-hearing unit—whether an academic department, a hospital clinic, or community freestanding clinic—is pyramidal in structure. It has a chairperson or director, perhaps an associate or assistant chair-

*Dr. Oyer is professor and director of Speech and Hearing Science, Department of Communication, The Ohio State University. He was formerly the chairman of the Department of Speech, Department of Audiology and Speech Sciences, and dean of the College of Communication Arts and Sciences at Michigan State University. He is Professor Emeritus of Audiology and Speech Sciences and Dean Emeritus of the Graduate School, Michigan State University.

person or director, some supervisors, etc. The formal authority and ultimate control generally reside with the principal administrator. This is not an unusual arrangement at all, for industrial, business, educational and religious organizations, for example, are similarly configured.

The literature dealing with organizational structure and managerial behavior is extensive. Theories of management are also plentiful, each resting upon a set of assumptions as to organizational structure, hierarchy of command, authority, task specialization, and division of staff and line responsibilities (McGregor, 1960). In McGregor's study of the managerial process, two management theories are described, one called *Theory X* and the other *Theory Y*.

Theory X maintains the traditional view of managerial direction and control. The assumptions that undergird it are that people dislike work, and that they must be directed and threatened with punishment if they are to produce results that help to achieve the objectives of the organization. Furthermore, the theory assumes that the average person prefers direction, has only little ambition, does not care for responsibility, and is interested in achieving security above all else.

Further consideration of the assumptions of Theory X, additional data, and recognition that direction and control approaches are of only limited value in motivating those whose needs supersede mere subsistence, led its originator to conclude that continued utilization of the assumptions of Theory X was often counterproductive. He suggests that as long as Theory X assumptions are influential in management, there will be a failure to discover and utilize people's full potential (McGregor, p. 43).

Although managers have made great strides in taking a more humane and enlightened approach to managerial strategy, Theory X assumptions continue to pervade managerial thinking. However, continued efforts to garner more data have led to the development of another set of assumptions, and eventually to a Theory Y (McGregor, p. 47-48). The assumptions are that effort expended in work is as natural as that expended in play or even at rest; that people will exercise self-direction and -control if they are committed to the objectives of the organization; that the extent to which people are committed to the objectives of the organization is in direct relation to the rewards they experience as a result of their achievements; and that the average person learns to accept as well as to look for responsibility. Furthermore, creativity in organizational problem solving is widely spread among employees and not a capacity that only few enjoy. Lastly, the intellectual potential of the average employee is only partially utilized. Thus, much intellectual power is going untapped. The organizing principle of Theory Y is that it is the integration of talents, skills, intellect, and the concepts of achievement of individual goals through effort that makes the enterprise successful. By contrast, the organizing principle of Theory X is that firm direction and control are the means by which the objectives of the organization can be met.

Not satisfied with the highly divergent views expressed by Theories X and Y, still another viewpoint has emerged, referred to as Theory Z (Barry, 1982). It assumes that the pyramidal organizational structure is here to stay, that there will continue to be a hierarchy of authority. However, in light of the impact of the human relations movement on managerial strategy, there is probably some point between Theories X and Y that represents an optimally realistic position. This blend of X and Y becomes Z. It supports the fact that some employees need more direction and control, whereas others produce with very little direction and control. Thus Theory Z suggests that within a Theory X organizational structure there is sufficient flexibility to permit the incorporation of the assumptions of Theory Y. Those not needing firm direction and control but who can realize self-fulfillment through working toward organizational goals are encouraged to do so.

Other theoretical positions have appeared which suggest managerial approaches to increased productivity. One such theory views the degree of individual maturation as being the key principle (Argyris, 1957), and suggests that there are seven steps involved as individuals develop from immature infants to mature adults. As maturation occurs there can be more reliance upon the individual to accomplish tasks. Research investigations support this contention.

Still another theoretical position is based on two concepts, motivation and hygiene (Herzberg et al., 1959). Herzberg's investigation showed that persons unhappy with their jobs were unhappy with the environment in which they worked; and that when people felt happy with their work it was on the basis of the work itself. Environment was defined broadly to include policies and administration, supervision, working conditions, interpersonal relations, money, status and security. Motivators were defined as achievement, recognition for accomplishment, challenging work, increased responsibility, and growth and development. Herzberg and colleagues found that improvement of environmental factors decreased dissatisfaction with the job but did not serve to motivate individuals to improve performance. However, they did find that satisfaction of the motivators permitted individuals to grow and mature and show increase in ability and performance.

Not a theory, but a summary of management systems, based on a study of organizations was offered by Likert (1967). The contention is that management styles are distributed along a continuum. *System-1* management shows no confidence or trust in subordinates and seldom involves them in decision making. Any informal organization that develops usually resists organizational goals. *System-2* depicts management as condescending toward lower-level employees and maintains control at the top. Any decision making that is delegated to lower levels is done so with condescension and reluctance, and is taken on with great caution and some discomfort by the subordinate. Informal organizations that develop are not necessarily always in opposition to formal organizational goals. *System-3* portrays management as being quite confident of the abilities of lower-level employees, and the latter are given substantial responsibility in decision making even though the broad policy-making functions are accomplished at the top. Some aspects of control are delegated downward and the informal organization that develops may at times resist goals of the organization. As one might expect, *System-4* is one in which management has complete confidence in the judgments of employees and trusts them implicitly. Communication is horizontal as well as vertical and the relationship between superiors and subordinates is collegial. Control is exercised by many individuals and the informal organization that develops is in effect no different from the formal organization, with both striving for success in meeting the objectives of the enterprise.

Not a theory, but more of a prescriptive approach to administration is advocated in a little story of a chief executive developed by Blanchard and Johnson (1982). They recognized the pyramidal structure in the story of the organization they describe, but also shaped the story so that it would qualify for a Theory Y setting or, in Likert's words, a System-4 organization, in which there is great confidence and trust in subordinates. Blanchard and Johnson refer to their approach as *The One-Minute Manager* and characterize the chief executive as one who expects his employees to succeed, and gives them every opportunity to do so. Important ingredients to success within this organizational style are goal setting, praise, and reprimands. In the goal setting there is agreement between superior and subordinate as to what those goals shall be; observation and identification of good behavior; writing down each goal in no more than 250 words; periodically reviewing the goals; spending a minute of each day looking at one's performance; and lastly determining whether or not one's goals and behaviors match. The praising works, according to the authors of this approach, when people are informed initially that they are going to be told how they are doing; people are praised immediately and are specifically told what they did right; people are emphatically told how good their superiors feel about their having done things right; and people are encouraged to do more of the same. According to the authors, the one-minute reprimand is as vital as goal setting and praising. They suggest that when a reprimand is in order it be given immediately, and employees informed as to what they did wrong and, after a few seconds have passed in silence, emphatically told how their superiors feel. They further suggest the reprimand be followed with a handshake and comments to let the employee know that he or she is supported and valued.

The ideas cited above represent what some theorists believe to be the fundamental assumptions that undergird management strategies as they are employed in the industrial and business communities. There is little question but that these assumptions have great relevance to the administration of speech-language and hearing programs. For such programs, in whatever setting and under whatever set of mandates they work, and with however many objectives, are units with similar structures to those found in business and industry. Similarly, they have personnel with individual needs and aspirations and differing levels of specialization and competency. Responsibilities are often specialized and there is a division of staff and line. Ultimately there is one who is in the seat of authority and must be held responsible for the decisions made within the unit. Although our speech-language-hearing units are pyramidal in structure with a head, chairperson, or director at the top, most of the decision making is done by group action. Thus the policy that guides the organization originates with those who will ultimately be responsible for the implementation of that policy. The principal reason that such an operation works is that speech-language-hearing units are composed of individuals who are similarly educated and for the most part share the same or at least similar professional values. Generally the speech-language-hearing unit is similar to the Likert System-4 approach to management, characterized by great confidence and trust vested in employees who exercise much of the policy making and control functions.

HEALTH INSURANCE

Developments over the past twenty years make it imperative that administrators responsible for providing speech-language pathology and audiology services become familiar with the insurance coverage to which their clients/patients are entitled. Insurance is provided to some extent by both private and public sources.

The Source Book of Health Insurance (1982-1983) contains interesting details of the relation between the magnitude of health expenditures and the gross national product. In the U.S. from 1960 to 1981 there has been a $259.7 billion increment in health expenditures. In 1960 national health expenditures comprised 5.3 percent of the gross national product as compared to 9.8 percent in 1981. According to the *Health Care Financing Review* (1983) private health insurance and other private third parties paid for 29.5 percent of the health costs in 1982 whereas government, via Medicare, Medicaid, and other federal, state and local programs supported 42.4 percent. Obviously the remainder, 28.1 percent came directly from patients themselves. Thus it is from these three general sources, namely, private insurance, government programs, and patient's direct payments, that funds are derived for services to patients with communicative disorders.

A superb treatment of the topic of health insurance as it pertains to speech-language pathology and audiology is provided in a manual published by the American Speech-Language-Hearing Association (Downey et al., 1984). The manual is aimed specifically at showing the reader the nature and rationale of both public and private health insurance programs, and how they cover patients with disorders of communication. It further suggests improvements in the coverage of communicative disorders and helps the reader to understand the coverage to which persons with disorders of communication are entitled. Furthermore, the manual is helpful in attempting advocacy for those not presently covered by any insurance programs.

The manual is the result of the efforts of a task force set up by ASHA in collaboration with several individuals within the ASHA National Office. The work of the task force was prompted by the requests the ASHA National Office received from members as to how greater access to services of speech-language pathology and audiology could be made available through health insurance. Considering the estimated 22 million persons in the United States who sustain disorders of communication, one can see why the topic is of more than passing interest to those responsible for administering programs of service.

When viewing the topic of health insurance as related to speech-language pathology and audiology services, one is impressed by the complexity of it all.

Which services can be reimbursed? How much can be expected for services rendered? How can services be contracted? How are claims made? What is the relationship with the physician in the collection of claims? How does one utilize supportive personnel? How do policies of Medicare differ from those of Medicaid? These issues are but a few of the many that swirl around the topic of health insurance in relation to payment of fees for services. These and others are discussed in the ASHA manual. The manual provides a tremendous source of information and should be especially useful to those who administer speech-language-hearing clinical programs.

ETHICS

Ethics deal with moral conduct, with matters of right and wrong. In codes of ethics developed and adopted by professional groups there are generally explicit and implicit principles given that undergird the proscriptions that follow.

Ethics are derived from values held by individuals, and codes of ethics are formalizations of those values shared by a group of individuals. Thus there are codes of ethics that "lay down the rules" in, for example, the practice of medicine, optometry, and dentistry. The American Speech-Language-Hearing Association (ASHA) maintains a code of ethics (Spahr, 1985–86) which has been carefully drafted to serve as a means of preserving high standards and integrity in those who engage as professionals in speech-language pathology and audiology.

There are six principles that the ASHA code of ethics embraces, including holding the welfare of persons served first and foremost; high standards of professional competence; accuracy of information provided by practitioners to the persons served and to the public regarding the nature and management of communicative disorders; maintaining objectivity in the delivery of service; honoring responsibilities to the public, the profession, colleagues, and members of allied professions; and lastly, upholding the dignity of the profession and accepting standards the profession has imposed upon itself.

Careful reading and occasional rereading of the ASHA code of ethics is indicated for all who engage in speech-language pathology and audiology, whether in practitioner or administrative capacity. However, administrators must be alert to the principles, proscriptions, and matters of professional propriety it provides not only for their own involvements but for all who serve professionally in any capacity within the program. Behavior that is not in compliance with the code of ethics can have profound implications not only for individuals but also for the programs they serve, irrespective of the setting. (See Appendix III for ASHA code of ethics.)

LEGISLATION

There is important legislation to be considered in the administration of speech-language-hearing units, regardless of their setting. The general concerns expressed by this legislation are for nondiscrimination, occupational health and safety, equal opportunity, affirmative action and due process. Individual states as well as the federal government have laws that must be adhered to. Some of the federal statutes are as follows:

Executive Order 11246.   Issued by the president of the United States in 1965 (Ex. Order) this statute places a requirement on all individuals who hold U.S. Government contracts or subcontracts to recruit affirmatively, hire, train, and promote minorities and women and to eliminate any discrimination in the employment of persons. Thus race, color, religion, national origin, and sex cannot be used as criteria in the selection or retention of employees. Periodic reviews of contractors are made by the U.S. Department of Labor to assure compliance.

Occupational Safety and Health Act of 1970.   The provisions of this act are most readily identified as *P.L. 91-596* (Occ. Safety and Health). The concern of this legislation is to assure that wherever individuals are at work, the environment is free of hazardous conditions that may affect their health and safety. The speech-language-hearing unit is generally not vulnerable to those hazards which can often be found in industry. Of particular professional interest to audiologists, however, is the hazard to hearing health caused by noise levels that are too high.

Amendment XIV.   As adopted July 21, 1868, Section 1 calls for protection of citizens' life, liberty, and property (Amend. XIV). No citizen shall be deprived of these "without due process of law." Due process implies the implementation of fair procedures before the State and its various public institutions can deny important interests of persons (Shrybman, 1982; Quirk, 1980). Although some procedures have become associated with due process, there is not a specific set of procedures associated with this concept. The procedures must be flexible enough to accommodate each situation that presents a new and different set of problems and considerations. With "fairness" as the central consideration, and proceedings that assure nonabridgement of individual rights, both the individual and the agency are setting the stage for well-conceived hearings, trials, and ultimately resolution of conflicts. Not only is the individual protected against unfair judgments but so is the agency. Although the basic principle of due process is within the Constitution, various court rulings and legislative actions have further defined the principle (Budoff and Orenstein, 1982). Administration of any program of speech-language-hearing must take into account the provisions of Amendment XIV.

The Older Americans Act of 1965 (P.L. 89-73).   This act provides assistance in the development of programs that help older people, including grants to states for training, research, and development. It was the most important legislation benefitting older people since the inauguration of the social security system in 1935. Groundwork for the Older Americans Act was laid in the deliberations and recommendations of the White House conference of 1961. The Older Amercians Act was responsible for the development of the Administration on Aging that has developed several programs. One program under Title III made grants to states for community service projects; another supported programs of research and demonstration under Title IV; the third supported training programs. The Administration on Aging has played a vital role in programming for older Americans since its beginnings.

The Age Discrimination In Employment Act of 1967 recognized that older Americans were being discriminated against in the workplace with mandatory retirement and replacement by advancing technology. In 1978 the act was substantially revised through the abolition of mandatory retirement for most federal employees and the increase to seventy the mandatory retirement age (Estes, 1979). Proper administration of speech-language-hearing programs takes into account the rights of older persons.

The Education of All Handicapped Children Act (Public Law 94-142). This act contains many provisions, with the major intent being that of assuring full and appropriate education to all handicapped children between the ages of three and twenty-one (Jones and Rabold, 1978). The act provides for safeguards for parents or guardians as well as for the children and professionals responsible for their education. Both speech-language pathology and audiology are included in the provisions of this law. Their inclusion has administrative implications for those responsible for overseeing programs involving communicatively disordered children. The federal law called upon each state to pass legislation responding to the P.L. 94-142 mandate (Rules for the Education of Hand. Child., Ohio Dep't. of Ed., 1982). It is of interest to note that local school systems can contract with community clinics to provide service, thus the provisions of the act become important in the administration of clinics that deliver services to the school system. The identification and evaluation of children with speech-language or hearing impairments, plus the development of the Individualized Education Program and its implementation with every child, have real implications administratively. Also, the establishment and implementation of the necessary due process safeguards are of genuine concern and call for administrative input and oversight (Crawford, 1978).

Rehabilitation Act of 1973 (P.L. 93-112), Section 504 "Nondiscrimination on the Basis of Handicap." This act was in a sense a civil rights law (Crawford, 1972). Section 504 specifies that no otherwise qualified person shall, on the basis of handicap, be denied benefits or be subjected to discrimination under programs receiving financial assistance. This applies to all citizens regardless of age. This law was generated in part because of the discrimination being felt by the handicapped Viet Nam war veteran. Section 504 carries a similar mandate as Title IX of the Education Admendments of 1972, which prohibits sex discrimination in most education programs receiving federal support. It reflects as well the mandate of Title VI of the Civil Rights Act of 1964 that prevents discrimination based on race or national origin (Goldberg, 1982).

Title VII of the Civil Rights Act of 1964 (Amended) (P.L. 88-352). This law has eleven titles and prohibits discrimination in employment because of race, national origin, color, religion or sex. Of particular importance are titles VI and VII. These deal with nondiscrimination in federally assisted programs and equal employment opportunity. Title III is also of importance to speech-language-hearing administrators as it deals specifically with desegregation of public facilities.

Title VII was amended by the Pregnancy Discrimination Act (P.L. 95-555) which prohibits sex discrimination on the basis of pregnancy. It provides pregnant women and those affected by childbirth or related medical conditions the same consideration as other employees not able to work.

Affirmative action and equal opportunity. Because society has long discriminated against minorities and women in its hiring practices, laws have been passed that require that *preference* be given to minorities and women in hiring and promotion. This is viewed as *affirmative action* (Silverman, 1983).

Affirmative action required, under the Equal Opportunity Act of 1972, that most federal contractors and subcontractors, as well as state governments and state institutions, develop and implement plans for increasing the number of women and minority employees (Squires, 1983). That no persons may be discriminated against because of race, color, sex, religion or national origin in being considered for employment is viewed as *equal opportunity*.

ACCREDITATION, CERTIFICATION, AND LICENSURE

The purpose of this section is to draw attention to other matters of legal concern that are relevant in the administration of speech-language-hearing programs. A matter of immediate administrative concern is that of program accreditation by the Educational Services Board (ESB, 1984) and the Professional Services Board (PSB, 1984) of the American Speech-Language-Hearing Association. Accreditation by ESB assures that institutions offering educational programs in speech-language pathology and audiology at the master's level meet minimal standards. Likewise, PSB accreditation assures that minimal standards are met in clinics delivering speech, language, and audiology services to the public. Full and complete instructions for accreditation review are available from the national office of the American Speech-Language-Hearing Association, 10801 Rockville Pike, Rockville, Maryland 20852.

Other matters of administrative concern are ASHA certification as well as licensure by states if such licensure exists. The certification of clinicians is through the American Speech-Language-Hearing Association. Applicants must present credentials that meet the academic, clinical practicum, and clinical fellowship year standards set forth by the association. The Certificate of Clinical Competence (CCC) is issued in both areas of speech-language pathology and in audiology. At the present time 35,876 hold the CCC in speech-language pathology, 5,337 in audiology, and 1,245 in both areas. The requirements for the Certificate of Clinical Competence are available in the ASHA *Directory* (Spahr, 1985–86).

Licensure, now required in 36 states, is another indication of the development of the profession. Once again individuals must certify that they possess the necessary credentials to practice speech-language pathology and/or audiology and qualify by passing the appropriate examination(s). The assurance to the state that licensing procedures are carried out properly is via the state licensing board. Licensure is required by states for the principal purpose of protecting the public from unqualified practitioners. Because of the necessity to define the activities of the practitioners, it also tends to exclude other professionals from involvement in those activities.

Accreditation, certification, and licensure, although of tremendous importance, constitute but three of the many issues with which the administrator must be familiar. Silverman presents in depth an excellent discussion of these and other issues such as malpractice, confidentiality, copyrights and patents, use of human subjects, lobbying, and presenting testimony as an expert witness (Silverman, 1982).

SUMMARY

Many concerns are inherent in the administration of speech-language-hearing units, the first of which is the way the unit will be administered. As we have seen, this can vary from relatively autocratic, to relatively democratic styles. Although the organization of the speech-language-hearing unit is usually pyramidal in configuration with a head, chair, or director, policy making and control functions are shared by many.

Health insurance plays a substantial role in health care delivery. As speech-language and hearing services are delivered, publicly supported health insurance plans through Medicare and Medicaid and privately funded insurance programs become important administrative concerns.

A code of ethics and legislation that govern the behavior of clinicians and patients are significant factors in the administration of speech-language and hearing units. The implications of legislation are far-reaching, including work environments, hiring, firing, and discrimination on bases of color, creed, sex, religion and age. The matter of due process is also of great importance to the administrative process. Rights of persons, including the handicapped, is also an imperative that must be observed.

Ethics, accreditation, certification and licensure are of genuine concern to administrators of speech-language and hearing programs. Such concerns attest to the responsibility borne by professionals at work in the field of communicative disorders.

REFERENCES

ACCREDITATION OF EDUCATIONAL PROGRAMS IN SPEECH-LANGUAGE PATHOLOGY AND AUDIOLOGY. (1984). *Educational standards board*. Rockville Pike: American Speech-Language-Hearing Association.

ACCREDITATION OF PROFESSIONAL SERVICE PROGRAMS IN SPEECH-LANGUAGE PATHOLOGY AND AUDIOLOGY. (1984). *Professional services board*. Rockville Pike: American Speech-Language-Hearing Association.

AMENDMENT XIV ADOPTED BY U.S. CONGRESS, JULY 21, 1969. *The Hammond almanac*. Maplewood, N.J.: Hammond Almanac, Inc., 80.

ARGYRIS, CHRIS. (1968). *Personality and organization*. New York: Harper and Row Publishers, Inc., 50.

BARRY, THOMAS J. (1982). "Theory X and theory Y in the organizational structure." Ph.D. diss., Southeastern University, ERIC Document 240693.

BLANCHARD, KENNETH, AND SPENCER JOHNSON. (1982). *The one minute manager* New York: William Morrow and Company, Inc., 34, 44, 59.

BUDOFF, MILTON, AND ALAN ORENSTEIN. (1982). *Due process in special education: On going to a hearing*. Cambridge, Mass: The Ware Press, 18.

CRAWFORD, WILLIAM L. (1978). *New help for the handicapped*. Toledo, OH: Lake State Printing Co., 27, 31.

DOWNEY, MORGAN, STEVEN C. WHITE, AND SUSAN KARR. (1984). *Health insurance manual for speech-language pathologists and audiologists*. Rockville, Md.: American Speech-Language-Hearing Association.

ESTES, CARROLL L. (1979). *The aging enterprise*. San Francisco: Jossey-Bass Publishers, 93.

EXECUTIVE ORDER 11246, *Weekly compilation of presidential documents*. September 24, 1965, 305–309.

GOLDBERG, STEVEN S. (1982). *Special education law*. New York: Plenum Press, 4.

HEALTH CARE FINANCING REVIEW. Fall, 1983 Vol. 5, No. 1. Source: Bureau of Data Management and Strategy, Health Care Financing Administration.

HERSEY, PAUL, AND KENNETH H. BLANCHARD. (1969). *Management of organizational behavior*. Englewood Cliffs, N.J.: Prentice-Hall, Inc., 42–57.

HERZBERG, FREDERICK, BERNARD MAUSNER, AND BARBARA SYNDERMAN. (1959). *The motivation to work*. New York: John Wiley, 113–119.

JONES, CLARENCE J. AND TED F. RABOLD. (1978). *Public law 94–142, a guide for the education for all handicapped children act*. State College, Pennsylvania: Penns Valley Publishers.

LIKERT, RENSIS. (1967). *The human organization*. New York: McGraw-Hill Book Co., 3–12.

MCGREGOR, DOUGLAS (1960). *The human side of enterprise*. New York: McGraw-Hill Book Company, Inc., 15, 43, 47, 48.

P.L. 91-596. OCCUPATIONAL SAFETY AND HEALTH ACT OF 1970. (1970–1971). *United States statutes at large*. 91st Congress, 2nd Session, Vol. 84, Part 2, 1590–1619.

P.L. 88-352 CIVIL RIGHTS ACT OF 1964. TITLE VII – EQUAL EMPLOYMENT OPPORTUNITY. (1964). *United States statutes at large*. 88th Congress, 2nd Session, 241–268.

P.L. 95-555 SEC. 701 OF THE CIVIL RIGHTS ACT OF 1964. PREGNANCY, SEX, DIS-CRIMINATION, PROHIBITION. (1978). *United States statutes at large*. 95th Congress, 2nd Session, 2076.

P.L. 89-73 OLDER AMERICANS ACT OF 1965. (1965). *United States statutes at large*. 89th Congress, 1st Session, 218–225.

QUIRK, JOHN P., Ed., (1980). *Readings in law and the execptional child: Due process*. Guilford, CT.: Special Learning Corporation.

RULES FOR THE EDUCATION OF HANDICAPPED CHILDREN. (1982). Columbus, Ohio: Ohio Department of Education.

SHRYBMAN, JAMES A. (1982). *Due process in special education*. Rockville, Md.: Aspen Systems Corporation, 3.

SILVERMAN, FRANKLIN H. (1983). *Legal aspects of speech-language pathology and audiology*. Englewood Cliffs, N.J.: Prentice-Hall, Inc., 146.

SOURCE BOOK OF HEALTH INSURANCE DATA. 1982–1983. Washington, D.C: Health Insurance Association of America.

SPAHR, FREDERICK T., Ed. *American Speech-Language-Hearing Association, 1985–86 Membership Directory, Code of Ethics*. Rockville, Md.: American Speech-Language-Hearing Association, xvii–xviii.

SPAHR, FREDERICK T., Ed. *American Speech-Language-Hearing Association, 1985–86 Membership Directory, Requirements for the Certificates of Clinical Competence*. Rockville, Md.: American Speech-Language-Hearing Association, xii–xxiii.

SQUIRES, GREGORY D. (1983). "Affirmative action." Academic American Encyclopedia. Danbury, CT.: Grolier, Inc., 132.

2 The Development of Speech-Language Pathology and Audiology in the United States

John J. O'Neill*

EUROPEAN INFLUENCES

The roots of the development of what was to become the speech and hearing profession in the United States are to be found in Europe during the nineteenth century. Rockey indicates that it was during that period that problems of communication were being differentiated and individuals were starting to join together to work in the area. Concern seemed to center on the management of speech and hearing disorders rather than on diagnosis or research, with the greatest interest directed towards the deaf. Geographical location was a crucial factor at this stage. Practitioners working on the Continent had medical backgrounds, whereas practitioners in Great Britain had backgrounds mainly in elocution.

In this review, four areas will be under consideration, those which appeared to be of interest at that time. All of the events described occurred well before any thought had been given to the development of a profession to deal with speech and hearing disorders.

The deaf. The first organized effort at managing a disorder of communication involved the deaf. In France a manual system was in vogue, while in Germany

*Dr. O'Neill is professor and former chairman of the Department of Speech and Hearing Sciences, University of Illinois. He is a past president of the American Speech-Language-Hearing Association.

13

an oral approach was advocated. Itard, in the early 1800s, reported on what appeared to be the first effort to use auditory training. Other individuals such as Blanchet and Deleau carried on the work after Itard's death. It involved training with changes in the intensity of bells and individual speech sounds. In the late 1800s Urbantschitsch in Germany reported on the use of auditory training with a deaf boy, and in 1895 he published a text on auditory training. There was a definite division between the manual and oral methods. The early work of del'Epee, which utilized the manual approach, was carried forth in France by Abbé Sicard, who developed a dictionary of signs, and by C. Deschamps and Ernaud. The oral method, the product of S. Heinicke, was initiated in Germany. The sites that demonstrated the two schools of thought were frequently visited by individuals from around the world, including several from the United States. In the British Isles Thomas Braidwood, a Scottish grammar school teacher, developed his own approach to teaching the deaf. Some individuals have indicated that the classifying of sounds by educators of the day in their efforts to develop remedial approaches led to the start of a new profession of speech correction.

Audiology. Major interest was in diseases of the ear rather than in the educational aspects of dealing with the hard of hearing. Most of the work in the area was being done by physicians who had received some specialized training in diseases of the ear. Two of these early physicians have been given the title "Father of Audiology" by several authors. These physicians were V. Urbanschitsch and F. Bezold. Both stressed the value of auditory training, but Bezold placed emphasis upon the significance of units of speech, as opposed to the individual sounds approach of Urbanschitsch. Tuning fork tests were developed to assist in the clinical diagnosis of hearing impairment. The Weber test developed in 1834 was one of the first of the qualitative hearing tests. It was followed by the Rinne test in 1885 which provided for a comparative evaluation of air conduction and bone conduction hearing. Very little was reported in regard to the development or use of the electric audiometer until two European investigators, A. Hartmann and D. E. Hughes, applied electric current to hearing tests. A. Politzer, one of the leading otologists in Europe at that time was quite optimistic about the possible use of such an instrument. In 1885 L. Jacobson added a second induction coil to the electric audiometer to control the intensity as well as the frequency of the tone. Also, several of the audiometers allowed for presentation of the tone by means of a hand-held telephone earphone.

However, the usual approach to hearing testing, if not with tuning forks, made use of such devices as the Galton-Edelman whistle or the monochord. Both of these devices presented tones that range in frequency from 4000 to 25,000 Hz. Individual sound amplification was accomplished through the use of the "ear trumpet" or speaking tube. These resonators were made of thin metal, brass, or vulcanite. The speaking tube allowed individuals to speak into a funnel at the end of the tube and the listener would insert the other end of the tube into the ear. Toynbee in

1862 was the first to conduct a histological investigation on ears with hearing damage.

Speech and voice disorders. In 1801 J. Thelwall in Great Britain indicated that he thought speech correction was a science as well as an art and the following were treating it as such. Dieffenbach, on the continent, was suggesting surgery of the tongue for stuttering and Broca and Wernicke were presenting their material on aphasias. Another continental practitioner, J. Muller, was in 1837 discussing the movement of the vocal folds, while M. Garcia developed the laryngeal mirror in 1854. H. Gutzman, Sr. and Albert Gutzman, his son, established the Berlin School for Speech and Voice Therapy and published numerous articles and books, while in Vienna R. Coen was recognized for his work with speech disorders. Charvin in France and Bell in Scotland were also considered to be experts in voice. Also in Great Britain, Hunt, in 1863, published a text on stammering and stuttering, and in 1894 a text on speech disorders was written by J. Wyllie. During the period from 1839 to 1894 there was in fact a veritable avalanche of textbooks dealing with stuttering and stammering. One of the problems of determining the significance of this work, especially in Great Britain, was the lack of scientific reports. Letters from eminent men served as a testimonial for the clinician, or patients rewarded the therapist with a portrait of themselves, and in one instance actually presented the therapist with a bust. During this period the concept of a profession was being developed, along with the determination of the problems with which it could deal. The point is made by Rockey that the battle over who should deal with stutterers assisted in determining that the area of speech correction should not become another medical specialty, and this gave further emphasis to the development of the independence of the profession.

Experimental phonetics or speech science. The first text to carry the title *Experimental Phonetics* was written by K. Rousselet in 1910. Even though research was quite limited some individuals were offering theories to explain certain speech phonemena. In 1830 W. Willis formulated what may have been the first scientific theory of vowel production. Several mechanical pieces of equipment were developed specifically for the study of the physical aspects of speech, including the spirometer developed by Hutchinson (1849), and the belt penumograph (1855) by H. Gutzman, Sr. The first stroboscopic observation of the larynx in 1878 was performed by M. J. Oertel and the first photographs of the larynx were produced by T. French in 1884. Most of the equipment made use of the pneumatic-mechanical principle which utilized levers, capsules and rubber tubes. This state existed until the principles of electricity were applied to the equipment.

Several other mechanical aids were being used during this period, including a tongue bridle or retractor, wooden plates shaped to the lower jaw, and the glossonochon tongue lever, which was a thin plate fastened to a lower tooth. H. von Helmholtz developed the resonators that carry his name to analyze tones (1913).

THE NINETEENTH CENTURY AND THE FIRST HALF
OF THE TWENTIETH CENTURY IN THE UNITED STATES

The European interest in speech and hearing provided a body of knowledge along with an orientation to the management of communication disorders that was carried to the United States. The education of the deaf attracted the earliest attention through the dedication of individuals who wanted to help deaf offspring or relatives. The only other area that attracted early attention was stuttering, which was discussed in medical texts or texts dedicated to training of the deaf. Simon suggests that in the twentieth century audiology and speech correction emerged as new professions to serve as an educational response to the developing public consciousness of the handicapped in the United States.

The early years. Representatives of what was still an undeveloped profession included Alexander Graham Bell, Thomas Gallaudet, E. W. Scripture and Walter Swift. Most of these individuals had visited experts or clinics in Europe where they either observed or received training in the methods espoused by specific individuals. In these early years there were no formal training programs, few clinics, and a fair amount of representation in the public schools. The early proponents had been trained as elocution teachers, physicians, and teachers of the deaf, while others were self-trained entrepreneurs.

The first recorded textbook on speech defects published in the United States has been attributed to S. C. L. Potter, who had practiced in Great Britain. Published in 1802, it carried the title *Speech and Its Defects*. In 1825 one of the first accounts of a private practice was attributed to a Mrs. E. Leigh. She utilized a method referred to as the Leigh Method, aimed at curing stuttering. Some authorities report that the method had been developed by a Dr. Yates who did not wish to have his name associated with it, so he used the name of his daughter's tutor. One account claims that Mrs. Leigh cured 150 people between the period 1828–1830. The early years were typified by the dogged use of "the method" associated with a particular master, but these methods were so closely guarded that there is not much information available in regard to them.

The speech disorder receiving the greatest attention was stuttering. Several physicians were using the surgical procedure developed by Dr. Diffenbach in Germany, which involved operations on the tongue of the stutterer. This was also the period of mechanical aids. For example, the aforementioned Mrs. Leigh suggested placing rolls of linen beneath the tongue during the hours of sleeping. This allowed the tongue to be in the "correct position" for speech with the tongue tip raised to the palate. Another approach involved the placing of a cork between the teeth.

The greatest service activity took place in the schools. Reports of such activity were made concerning the Grand Rapids schools (107 children in the period between 1916–1917) and the Chicago, Detroit, Minneapolis and New York school systems. In 1922 a survey undertaken in Wisconsin indicated that some nineteen hundred children, or 5 to 7 percent of the students surveyed, needed speech help.

Another survey in St. Louis indicated that 5.7 percent of the children in the public and parochial schools required speech assistance. Of some interest is the title of an article that appeared in a 1917 issue of a medical journal, "The Economic Value of Speech Correction." The concept of cost effectiveness is not so new! The article further indicated that speech defects should be treated as soon as the child entered school. Some four years later Smiley Blanton reported on a psychoneurotic type of speech disorder which was related to a wartime experience. Also, at about the same time the first commercially available manual for the correction of speech defects appeared from a medical book publisher. The White House conference of 1930 estimated that among children between the ages of five and eighteen there were one million requiring remedial speech treatment. Also, it was recommended that every school system should have school programs in speech correction.

The Martin Institute for Speech Correction was in operation in Ithaca, New York in 1926, while the Boston Stammerers Institute had been in operation in Boston since 1867. Speech clinics were in operation from 1916 at the University of Wisconsin, from 1928 at Northwestern University, at the New York University medical school in 1925 and Washington University in 1926. In 1936 the first issue of the *Journal of Speech Disorders* appeared and in 1931 one of the first textbooks in the field, *Speech Pathology* by L. Travis, appeared. Ten years before, the first meeting of the National Society for the Study and Correction of Speech Disorders was held. In New York the National Hospital for Speech Disorders was established by members of the so-called Viennese School, including such individuals as Froeschels and Weiss. The first formal laboratory for research in speech science, the Flo Brown Memorial Laboratory, was established at the University of Wichita in 1935. Other laboratories associated with academic training programs were developed in the 1920s and 1930s at the University of Iowa and Ohio State University. A thesis dealing with the experimental analysis of causes of stuttering was submitted in 1921 at the University of Wisconsin and in 1924 there was a listing of two theses in speech pathology at the University of Iowa. The first reported effort at speech correction at the college level appeared in 1923 in the *Quarterly Journal of Speech* and was written by Sara Stinchfield in regard to the student population at Mt. Holyoke College. She reported that 17 percent of the student population required some corrective work. Classes in speech improvement were initiated at Smith College in 1922 and administered by the Spoken English Department. Of some historical interest was the following reported faculty additions in 1936: Charles Van Riper joined the staff at Western State Teachers College at Kalamazoo and John W. Black became the head of Speech at Kenyon College. In 1934 Raymond Carhart completed a thesis that dealt with the study of the relation between cushion pipes and subglottic resonators.

Audiology.   The pure tone audiometer came into its own in the United States. The first vacuum tube audiometer was developed in 1921, and the first commercial model was the Western Electric 1A, the brainchild of Dr. Edmund Fowler, an otologist. It was a nonportable unit and its cost ($1,500) was viewed as excessive. Other audiometers were introduced by other manufacturers. Included were the Sonotone unit developed by Jones and Knudsen and a unit developed by Kranz. These units tested the frequency range from 32 to 16, 384 d.v. (Hz in present language) and higher. The difficulty with these models was that none of them used a universally accepted reference level and the intensity units were labeled as sensation units rather than decibels. The Council on Physical Therapy of the American Medical Association, in conjunction with the American Standards Association, in 1937–1939 established standards for audiometers in terms of frequency and intensity ranges, including five decibel steps. In 1937 the Maico D-5 audiometer was introduced. This was the first audiometer with a zero reference level that was adjusted automatically for each frequency. The first articles that dealt with the design of soundproofed rooms appeared in the professional literature in 1938. One of the greatest breakthroughs in terms of diagnostic audiology occurred when the two-channel audiometer was developed. This development allowed the audiologist to have separate control over the intensity of the stimulus for each channel.

Hearing aids.   The electric hearing aid came about through the development of the telephone by Alexander Graham Bell. The first such hearing aid was of the carbon variety, in which the movement of electrically charged carbon granules made it possible to transfer sound to electrical charges which varied with changes in the frequency and intensity of the speech. Berger writes that the first carbon hearing aid was developed by M. R. Hutchinson in 1899. The carbon aid proved to be impractical because of its size and the distortion and noise in the microphone, but nevertheless it was the instrument of choice until the late 1930s. After World War II, with the advent of the vacuum tube, it became possible to have more reliable and accurate amplification of sound. With the advent of the printed circuit and the development of the transistor it became possible to make the hearing aid smaller. Along with this reduction in the size of the instrument came a decrease in battery size.

Auditory training units.   The first electrical, group auditory training unit, named the Electrophone, appeared in 1921. Another unit, the Acuovox, was developed about the same time. It enabled students to hear their own voices and the voices of the other students and the teacher as well. The first group auditory training unit was developed by Currier and consisted of multiple conversation tubes so that five students could be trained at one time. In the same reference Goldstein also described the CID multiple tube unit, which enabled larger groups of youngsters to receive auditory stimulation at one time. From 1930 to 1935 individual as well as multiple nonwearable vacuum tube group auditory training units were being placed in leagues for the hard of hearing, churches, and schools for the deaf. Several of the major hearing aid manufacturers, especially Maico, started to develop commercially available auditory training units in the 1950s. The development of such units can be attributed to the tremendous reception given to the organized auditory programs developed at the Deshon and Hoff general army hospitals as part of the armed services aural rehabilitation programs. The majority of the amplification equipment used in the army-sponsored AR programs were specially constructed for use in the programs. The early commercial units incorporated these electronic developments into the units that were being presented for sale. Shortly after the beginning of the 1950s some seven to eight companies were selling commercial auditory training units. Three of these companies (Maico, Warren and Grason Stadler) were still manufacturing units at the end of the 1970s. In the 1960s loop units and, later, radio frequency units were developed. These developments enabled teachers to avoid the hard wire features which had restricted the mobility of teacher and pupils.

Speech reading. The development of speech reading in the United States took three directions: the importing of a method developed in Europe, the development of a new method, and the expansion of the newly developed method. The Mueller-Walle approach was brought to Boston by Martha Bruhn, a hard-of-hearing individual who had taken a six-week course from J. Mueller-Walle in Germany. She translated the method into English and opened a school of lipreading in Boston. Another method that was brought to this country was the Jena method. This method, developed by Brauckmann, used a motor as well as visual approach to the teaching of lipreading. It was translated and expanded by several individuals at the University of Michigan, the best known of the group being Anna Bunger of Eastern Michigan University. Her name became associated with this approach.

One of the first individuals to develop her own method in this country was Lillie Warren, who dealt with an analytic system that assigned numbers to sixteen "visible" sounds. She established the first speech reading classes in the United States. One of her students, Edward Nitchie, in 1903 wrote a book on self-instruction in lipreading which Warren claimed was plagiarized from her method. Over the next twenty years Nitchie's approach became a more synthetic one and he and his wife published some four or five texts in the area, the basic approach involving drills with syllables. The Kinzie sisters, Cora and Rose, developed their own school of speech reading in Philadelphia in 1917. Their method was a combination of elements from the Mueller-Walle methods and the Nitchie approach. Another method developed during this early period was that of Louise M. Morgenstern, and consisted of a series of lessons utilizing sounds as well as conversational materials. These materials were used in evening classes in the public schools in New York. In 1915 the Cincinnati Board of Education authorized evening lipreading classes. An article in a 1914 issue of the *Laryngoscope* described a program which involved two or three lipreading lessons a day and indicated that the students learned lipreading in a period of two months. Also, during this same period an article entitled Ear and Aviation appeared in, of all places, the *Archives of Neurology and Psychiatry*. In 1926 the first school screening program was undertaken in New York with the 4A audiometer. The investigators indicated that through screening in the schools cases would appear other than those present at the physician's office. In 1935 Robert West pushed the idea of developing hearing aids which would have the effect upon hearing that corrective lenses had upon vision. Also, he indicated that the aids should be light in weight, compact, inconspicuous and dependable. He further indicated that he felt deafness was a problem of lack of range as well as a lack of acuity. West had developed a test for the evaluation of hearing aids that made use of words that carried specific frequency characteristics. In this early period an individual who was later to be heavily identified with speech disorders was providing some of the most innovative ideas about hearing aids.

At the end of the 1940s the profession was receiving attention for its service activities. Along with the development of sophisticated instrumentation, this resulted in the development of speech and hearing clinics, which in turn necessitated the assignment of administrative responsibilities. Thus the early members of the profession were beginning to obtain exposure to administrative roles.

POST WORLD WAR II PERIOD

In the discussion that follows the events that occurred during the profession's most formative years are described. When one views the situation immediately after the conclusion of World War II, the speech-language pathology and audiology profession was shaped by seven factors. These factors were: change in professionals outlook and orientation; increases in federal funding; growth of the national professional organization; development of academic autonomy; national and state legislation; expansion of service activities; and increases in training programs.

Change in professional outlook and orientation. The period immediately after the war was typified by a tremendous increase in funds for higher education through the GI Bill of Rights, with a resulting increase in the availability of postsecondary education. Also, some individuals gained experience during the war working in the newly developed rehabilitation centers, plus a sense of idealism, and thus had an orientation toward the treatment of handicaps, including severe communication difficulties. One small group of individuals in particular, who had gained extensive and intensive experience working in interprofessional environments, had witnessed the successful results of short-term, intensive therapy as well as the efficacy of treating the "whole man."

Increases in federal funding. Along with such changes in orientation at the professional level came increases in funding at the federal level. In 1943 the United States Congress had indicated that the Veterans Administration should be the agency in charge of all service-connected rehabilitation programs. Between 1943 and 1948 there was a pronounced increase in the number of speech and hearing rehabilitation programs being conducted both in Veterans Administration hospitals and through contracts with college or university speech and hearing clinics. Some funding had been available since 1949, when the Children's Bureau provided funds for service programs and traineeships at Johns Hopkins University. In 1950 similar funding was provided at the University of Iowa. Also, financial assistance for services was provided through two of the subunits of the agency, the Maternal and Child Health and Services for Crippled Children units.

The first federal agency to provide extensive funding for speech and hearing training programs was the Vocational Rehabilitation Administration, located in the U.S. Department of Health, Education and Welfare. The agency had received authorization for such training activities, as well as for research and demonstration activities, through the Vocational Rehabilitation Act Amendments of 1954 (Public Law 565, 83rd Congress.) Then, between 1963 and 1974, the time was very ripe for the development of the profession, as Flower indicates, in that the federal government had made a unique commitment to the development of human services through the passage of certain items of legislation. In 1966, as part of the "Great Society" activities of the Lyndon Johnson administration, the Bureau of Education for the Handicapped was formed, resulting from an amendment to the Elementary and Secondary Education Act of 1965 (Public Law 89-10). These various funding activities allowed for the growth of master's level training in speech and hearing. In 1965 at perhaps the peak of such activity, the VRA funds were allocated to some sixty six training programs. This support probably provided the greatest impetus for the growth of the profession, through the increase in opportunities for training it offered. The Office of Education provided $1,229,300 for training, as contrasted to the $8,500,000 provided by VRA.

While doctoral training programs received some funding from the previously mentioned two sources, the greatest support for this level of training came from the National Institutes of Neurological Disease and Stroke, with some additional assistance from the National Institute of Dental Research. Since the mid-1960s sufficient training funds were available to encourage more individuals to select the discipline for graduate study. With the beginning of the 1970s, however, there was a decrease in funding for training. This decrease has continued until the present day, with approximately twenty-five to thirty graduate programs having federal funding. Also, the NIH institutes dropped funding for predoctoral training in speech pathology and audiology.

Growth of national organization. The growth in funding described above can be attributed in part to the tenor of the times, but it can also be attributed to the establishment of a national office of the American Speech and Hearing Association in Washington, D.C. and later in Bethesda, Maryland. This organization began assembling and disseminating statistics about the operations of the professions as well as serving as an advocate at the United States Congress. In the fall of 1959 the association introduced the journal *Asha*, which served as its house organ and became the source for much of the data about the profession, with the presentation of the results of surveys, position papers, proposals for changes in organization, certification, federal legislation, and professional events.

The findings of the first survey published in the journal is of interest. The results included the following: Twenty-five institutions had OVR (Office of Vocational Rehabilitation—the original name of the Rehabilitation Services Administration) grants and there were forty training programs at the masters level and thirty at the doctoral-masters level. In the same year (1959) Kenneth Johnson, executive secretary of the organization, indicated that there were several major issues facing the profession. Two of the more important dealt with the need for developing independence, along with the need to develop a professional identity. Beginning in 1965 ASHA started to accredit training programs in speech pathology and audiology as a result of negotiations with the National Council on Accreditation, the American Medical Association, and the American Dental Association. The accreditation program had been initiated in 1961 with the formation of the American Boards of Examiners in Speech Pathology and Audiology, under whose direction two boards were in operation. These were the Education and Training Board and the Professional Services Board, with the latter being responsible for the accreditation of service or clinic programs. Over the past twenty years there has been a continuing argument as to whether clinics associated with training programs should be accredited. There have been surges of pro and con activities, and as of 1983 there were 258 clinical facilities accredited by the Professional Services Board with forty-four of them being university speech and hearing clinics.

The national organization continues to be quite active as, for example, the accrediting agency for master's degree programs in speech pathology and audiology; as an advocacy and public information unit for the profession; serving in a lobbying role; developing a standards program; and providing services to state associations and individual members.

Development of academic autonomy.   As was indicated earlier, the discipline did not show signs of gaining departmental status until the 1950s. Before then the operation of training programs was usually under the direction of the individual who was serving as head of the speech department. In the early 1900s the discipline of speech was a part of English departments under the rhetoric section. Around 1915 the first of the speech units left English and developed departments of rhetoric or speech. As of 1915 there were some fourteen state universities with separate departments of speech, with six being in the Midwest. There were few courses to be taught in the area of speech and hearing disorders in the early years, and the only function that could bring an individual some status or academic identification was serving as head of a speech and/or hearing clinic—if the individual's institution condoned remedial services. Once such a clinic was available and services were being provided it became obvious that additional trained individuals were needed to work with disorders of communication. Simon writes that the pattern of the university clinic serving as a training center had been very well established in some areas before World War I, but it did not appear that very many such clinics were in operation until after World War II. As funding for training increased and as national certification came into full bloom, along with an increase in the funds for service, a faculty member trained in the speech pathology and audiology area was probably directing a clinic, teaching courses, obtaining training funds, doing some clinical supervision, and acting as head of a section within a speech department. Also, because of the need for clinic and laboratory space, a physical separation may have developed from colleagues in the speech department and attention was turned to possible affiliation with medicine, special education or in some instances psychology.

The eventual move toward departmental status can be attributed to several causes. The first involved the "follow-the-leader" syndrome. As the programs in the major universities started to establish departmental status others scrambled to follow their example. Also, ASHA started to stress certification requirements that called for speech and hearing personnel in academic settings to have greater freedom to establish academic requirements. It is difficult to establish a date when departmental status occurred for the majority of the profession. Some of the delay in establishing departments could be attributed to academic inertia, to campus politics and in some instances to philosophical disagreements.

In 1959 Carhart proposed that speech pathology and audiology should be considered as an independent educational field dealing with the social and educational aspects of communicative breakdowns. Four years later, Peterson and Fairbanks authored an article that included among its several viewpoints a conclusion that the profession had the necessary academic material for a separate discipline, which they thought should be called *speech and hearing science*. Cluff reported that the majority of his respondents in a national survey indicated that departmental status allowed them to obtain professional recognition, and facilitated growth. In the large university or college setting the speech and hearing department is usually viewed as a small to medium unit. In the smaller colleges or universities the department may be viewed as one of the larger but also as one of the stronger departments. From the results of a 1984 survey undertaken by the National Council of Graduate Programs in Speech-Language Pathology and Audiology it appears that 45 percent of the responding departments were located in Arts and Sciences settings, 22 percent in Education settings, and 16 percent in Health and Medicine settings. As heads of departments, members of the profession served on the usual university committees, were actively involved in college matters, and obviously did not disgrace their lineage. In fact, some did such an excellent job that they were appointed deans. In the past few years at least six have served as deans of graduate schools, several more as deans of colleges of Applied or Affiliated Health and Humanities, Social Sciences and Education, and Communication Arts and Sciences. At least three have become university presidents. If individuals serve as a head of a department they may have to wear another hat as director of a speech and hearing clinic. In any event they find there is a need to satisfy a variety of masters.

What roles do members of these relatively new departments play? Muma et al. reported that a high percentage of such faculty members carried large clinical loads and were not very involved in research or community service. Also, senior clinical staff members viewed administration as the least demanding of their activities, under training, clinical service, and research, in that order.

National and state legislation.   One of the major reasons for the growth of a profession is its acceptance by the professional community. This acceptance is usually evidenced by certification or licensure laws. Of key importance to the profession was the acceptance by accreditation agencies of the certification pattern developed by ASHA. Because the public schools utilized a large number of members of the profession, the initial battle began with state certification. The national organization representing the profession operated from the desire to develop its own standards for certification rather than have standards forced upon it. The resulting difficulties could be attributed in part to the fact that the profession was attempting to interfere with other professions that had not developed the type of certification standards that we had through ASHA.

A second area involved federal legislation which provided funding for training. With regard to the Vocational Rehabilitation Administration, the funding was for graduate training towards a masters degree. Other professional disciplines involved in such training included rehabilitation counseling, social work, and public health. Thus the pattern of training, and the resulting certification requirements for persons working in rehabilitation settings, was greatly influenced by this federal funding. One other item of federal funding that provided for the setting of minimal requirements was the legislation known as the Social Security Act, especially titles XVIII and XIX, which developed the plans for Medicare and Medicaid. Amendments to the act provided funding for speech pathology services. Also, the requirements indicated that the minimal level of training required for persons to be reimbursed for services were basically those specified in the ASHA certification requirements. These pieces of legislation, along with the requirements of Public Law 94-142, which extended public education down to age three years, not only brought the significance of services in speech-language and hearing to the attention of the public, but also provided funding which in turn expanded the job market. In the private sector the spinoff from the federal legislation resulted in many insurance companies authorizing payment for speech pathology services and some audiology services.

With the increase in funding came pressures for licensures. The ASHA certification system was not viewed by governmental or service groups as sufficient to cover the legal difficulties that went along with such funding. The first state licensure law was approved in 1969 in Florida. As of 1986 thirty-six states have licensure in speech pathology and audiology. In all but one or two states the licensure requirements are equivalent to the ASHA certification requirements. Thus, it is possible to obtain reciprocity among the majority of the states. There is some developing skepticism about the value of licensure. This is due to the confusion over the possible licensure of speech and hearing personnel in the schools.

Academic training. While speech correction was in operation in the public schools in the early 1900s, no official training programs came into operation until the 1930s. The early professionals either received their training in Europe, were trained in the general area of speech, or were dedicated classroom teachers serving in a specialized capacity. In 1916 the newly developed department of speech at the University of Illinois included a section on speech science that offered courses such as phonology, phonetics, psychology of audition, physics of sound, and physiology of the voice. In 1916 an article that appeared in the *Journal of Educational Psychology* indicated that the University of Wisconsin was training teachers for speech correction work in the schools. In the same article there was a statement to the effect that teachers should know the anatomy and physiology of the speech mechanism and they should learn to detect speech defects, especially in the lower grades. In a 1933 report in the *Quarterly Journal of Speech* there was an indication that 27.6 percent of the colleges in the United States offered facilities for a major in speech correction and that 28.9 percent had a clinic. In 1923 the University of Wisconsin catalogue contained the listing of a course in the correction of speech disorders. A later report indicated that in 1936 four universities offered courses in speech and hearing therapy. In the mid-1930s a survey of the first twenty years of the *Quarterly Journal of Speech* revealed that 7 percent of the publications were in the area of speech correction and that authors from four schools in the Midwest were the most prolific publishers. The schools were the universities of Illinois, Iowa, Michigan and Wisconsin. In a speech before the National Association of Teachers of Speech in 1933 J. M. O'Neill, the past president of the group, said that there were signs of disintegration in the group because of the desires for separation by staff members in the areas of speech correction and theatre. The late 1930s and early 1940s saw what Paden described as the beginning of the growth of a profession concerned with disorders of communication. In 1925 the American Academy of Speech Correction was founded. That group went through several name changes and in 1947 adopted the name *American Speech Correction Association*. It was now possible for an academic program to represent a nationally recognized discipline. The period from 1950 through 1960 saw the period of greatest growth, as was described under the section dealing with funding.

As a sign of its growing maturity, members of the profession held a conference on graduate education in 1963 with the intent of defining long-term goals of the profession as well as providing suggestions for a curriculum in graduate education. Several key points emerged from the many resolutions adopted at the conference. They were to serve as guiding beacons for the next ten to fifteen years. There was a strong emphasis upon the need for training programs to be located in a liberal arts and science setting. Also, the training program should have a core of training that centered around such areas as basic communicative processes, human growth and development, phonetics, and speech and hearing science. In 1983 a second national conference on graduate education was held. The concern of the conference was broadened to include consideration of undergraduate and continuing education. Many of the recommendations that resulted from that conference echoed those of the 1963 meeting. Several additional resolutions dealt with such areas as specialty training, the need to strengthen the theoretical and scientific bases of graduate education, as well as to strengthen the role of research. As Rees indicated in her summary of the conference, the key points were the support of the concept of a discipline, and the reaffirmation of the master's degree as the minimal preparation level. In 1976 the training programs in the "big ten" held a conference to discuss the professional doctorate, with the net result that little support existed for such a degree. In 1978 the directors of graduate training programs formed a national group, the Council on Graduate Programs in Speech-Language Pathology and Audiology. This group has held five annual conferences to deal with topics of immediate interest. It has changed its name to the National Council of Graduate Programs in Communication Disorders and Sciences. This change reflects the group's efforts to develop a common title for the profession.

Service activities.   Clinical services in both speech pathology and audiology had been fairly well established prior to 1945 both as independent clinical settings and as ancillary services in various types of medical settings. Speech pathology had been well established in some public schools since 1917. Because of the development of certification requirements in most states after 1950, speech pathology services became established more extensively in public schools. Audiology, however, except in Indiana and Utah, had not up to this date developed a certification requirement that allowed it to be involved in activities in the schools. Relationships between audiologists and educators of the deaf were still strained despite the fact that a national conference was held in Tucson in 1964 followed by nine regional conferences for the purpose of developing better relationships. As a result of the aforementioned difficulties in the schools situation, audiology was more likely to be involved in medical settings and community clinics. According to an ASHA survey published in 1965, 84 percent of the members were involved in providing clinical or educational services, with 56 percent involved in services in the schools.

In the 1960s there was a developing interest in language disorders, early work in the diagnosis of such disorders being reported by W. Hardy, H. Myklebust and S. Kastein. This early interest, along with contacts with linguists and the growth of the Chomsky "wave," lead more and more training and service programs to include course work and services in the area of language. In 1980 there was a move to develop special certification for a language clinician. This move led in turn to a review of the concept of single certification, and there was considerable discussion over the role members of the profession could play in the area of language learning difficulties, auditory processing difficulties, and learning disabilities. In some states speech and language clinicians were doing clinical work with children with learning difficulties, while in other states learning disabilities specialists were working with children with speech and language difficulties. Several members of the profession, including J. Eisenson, B. Porch, H. Schuell and J. Wepman, had been interested for many years in the language disorders of adults, as typified by aphasia. This interest had carried over from programs for brain-damaged veterans of World War II, and several of the most popular tests of aphasia had been developed by W. Halstead, J. Wepman, J. Eisenson and H. Schuell. Also, early research with language disorders associated with mental retardation had been undertaken in a large-scale project at Parsons Hospital and the University of Kansas by R. Schiefulbusch and his colleagues. Several of the individuals trained as part of the project assumed leadership positions in the area of language disorders.

Many of the textbooks published during the 1970s concentrated on the areas of language development, language disorders, and language evaluation. With this increased interest in language the service market received another stimulus. Then, with the development of service possibilities in audiology, came the development of certain types of instrumentation. In the 1950s the galvanic skin testing unit was popular because of Veteran's Administration testing requirements. Later on in the late 1950s and the early 1960s Bekesy audiometry became the test of choice for more sophisticated evaluation. This was assisted by the issuance of the Jerger typology for Bekesy tracings. The next stage of equipment development involved impedence testing, electronystagmography, and evoked response. With each improvement in equipment, audiology became more sophisticated in terms of its testing capabilities.

Speech pathology, on the other hand, was not quite as involved with the development of new equipment. There were certain pieces of equipment that proved to be valuable for assistance in diagnostic testing in certain areas: cineradiographic testing for cleft palate patients, pneumotachography for air flow measures, and strain gauges to measure lip and jaw movements. In essence speech pathology was more involved in the development of therapy techniques and clinical materials than with diagnostic activities.

The period between 1937 and 1948 witnessed tremendous progress in hearing aid development. The distortion in hearing aids was reduced, the frequency range was extended and the overall output of the aid was improved. The continuing argument over selective fitting was somewhat alleviated by the issuance of the often mentioned Harvard report in 1945. This report indicated that a high frequency emphasis on the order of 3 to 6 decibels would accommodate most hearing losses. Then the eyeglass hearing aid appeared and in the early 1960s the CROS and BICROS aids were introduced and in 1964 behind-the-ear hearing aids were first introduced.

During the 1950s audiology became quite active in terms of evaluation of individuals with suspected otosclerosis. The results of pure tone, speech reception, and discrimination tests were used in selecting candidates who would be successful candidates for surgery. One of the better known audiological characteristics developed during this period was the Carhart notch.

The concept of electrical activity in the brain was first reported in 1875, and in this country P. Davis in 1939 was the first investigator to report on the evoked response, as Brazier writes. In the later part of 1950 several individuals became involved with evoked response testing, and Clark in 1958 at MIT developed the average response computer.

Also, during the period of the late 1950s came the building of individual clinic units, which set a pattern for future units. They were developed at Gallaudet College, the Bill Wilkerson Center in Nashville, and the Cleveland Hearing and Speech Center.

The area of private practice has not developed to the extent some individuals might have liked. In 1961 ASHA devoted one issue of the journal *Asha* to the discussion of private practice. The report had been prepared by the ASHA committee on private practice. At about the same time the American Academy of Private Practice in Speech Pathology and Audiology was formed. In 1981 A. Feldman in his presidential address stressed the need for professional autonomy and the need for expansion of the profession into the private sector.

Present status and concerns. The present status of the profession can be detailed, to some degree, by glancing at the topics under consideration at annual conferences and by studying the resolutions that arise from those conferences. In general, it would appear that the items of concern for the 1980s reflect the problems of the time. In the academic area the concern is, as always, with the recruitment of quality students, and also with the nature of a "core" curriculum, supervision of clinical practicum, the academic status of the supervisor, and the need for a continuing scientific approach to the concerns of the profession. In the service area, concerns are for the effects of decreased funding upon human services; the role of the speech-pathologist and audiologist (since it appears they serve as supporting professionals within both educational and medical settings, rather than as independent decision makers); the need for growth in the area of private practice; and the continuing distance between clinical problems and research interests.

Members of the profession as well as the national organization have become quite active in regard to federal legislation. At the state level, committees or individuals have been assigned the task of staying current with and influencing ongoing legislative activities that may have an impact on the profession.

The profession has exhibited considerable growth in just over fifty years. It still appears to be growing and to be facing clinical and academic problems. Appropriate solutions may enable it to enjoy further growth.

REFERENCES

BERGER, KENNETH W. (1974). *The hearing aid: Its operation and development*. Livonia, Mich.: National Hearing Aid Society.

BRAZIER, MARY A. B. (1984). "Pioneers in the discovery of evoked potentials," *Electroencephalography and Clinical Neurophysiology*, 59, #1, 2–8.

BUNCH, C. C. (1943). *Clinical audiometry*. St. Louis. Mo.: C.V. Mosby, chapter 9.

CARHART, RAYMOND. (1960). "Speech pathology and audiology," *Asha*, 2, 99–102.

CLUFF, GORDON L. (1970). "Pros and cons of departmentalization—A survey of college and university speech pathology and audiology programs," *Asha*, 11, 557–559.

COUNCIL OF GRADUATE PROGRAMS IN COMMUNICATIVE SCIENCES AND DISORDERS. *1983–84 National Survey*.

CURTIS, JAMES F. (1954). "The rise of experimental phonetics." In *History of Speech Education in America*. Ed. Karl R. Wallace. New York: Appleton-Century-Crofts, chapter 16.

DICARLO, LOUIS M. (1964). *The deaf*. Englewood Cliffs, N.J.: Prentice-Hall, Inc.

FELDMAN, ALAN. (1981). "The challenge of autonomy," *Asha*, 12, 941–945.

FLOWER, RICHARD M. (December 1983). "Keynote address: Looking backward and looking forward: Some views through a four-decade window." In *Proceedings of the 1983 Conference on Undergraduate, Graduate and Continuing Education*. Ed. Norma S. Rees and Trudy L. Snope. *ASHA Reports 13*.

FROESCHELS, EMIL, (1962). "A survey of European literature in speech and voice pathology," *Asha*, 4, 172–181.

GOLDSTEIN, MAX A. (1933). *Problems of the deaf*. St. Louis, Mo.: Larynogoscope Press.

LUCHSINGER, RICHARD, AND GODFREY E. ARNOLD, eds. (1965). *Voice-speech-language. clinical communicology: Its physiology and pathology.* Belmont, Calif.: Wadsworth Publishing Co.

MOELLER, DOROTHY. (1976). *Speech pathology and audiology.* Iowa City, Iowa: U. of Iowa.

MOORE, PAUL, AND DOROTHY G. KESTER. (1953). "Historical notes on speech correction in the pre-association era," *JSHD*, 18, 48–53.

MUMA, JOHN R., MARY B. MANN AND SARAH A. TRENHOLD. (1976). "Training programs in speech pathology and audiology: Demographic data, perceived departmental and personal functions, and productivity," *Asha*, 18, 419–432 and 445–446.

PADEN, ELAINE P. (1970). *History of the american speech and hearing association, 1925–1958.* Washington, D.C.: American Speech and Hearing Association.

PETERSON, GORDON E. AND GRANT FAIRBANKS, (1963). "Speech and hearing science," *Asha*, 5, 539–543.

REES, NORMA S. (December 1983). "Summary and implications" in *Proceedings of the 1983 Conference on Undergraduate, Graduate and Continuing Education.* Ed. Norma S. Rees and Trudy L. Snope. *ASHA Reports 13.*

ROCKEY, DENYSE. (1980). *Speech disorder in nineteenth-century Britain.* Croom-Helm, 13.

SCHOOLFIELD, LUCILLE D. (1938). "The development of speech correction in America in the nineteenth century," *Quarterly J. of Speech*, 24, 101–116.

SIMON, CLARENCE T. (1954). "Development of education in speech and hearing to 1920." In *History of Speech Education in America.* Ed. Karl R. Wallace. New York: Appleton-Century-Crofts, chapter 18.

URBANTSCHITSCH, VICTOR. (1982). *Auditory training for deaf mutism and acquired deafness.* Trans. S. Richard Silverman. Washington: Alexander Graham Bell Association for the Deaf, Inc.

3 Some Reflections on Leadership

D. C. Spriestersbach*

There is an extensive literature on the subject of leadership, and I have read a small sample of it since accepting this assignment. That reading has been helpful in giving my experiences context and perspective. But this discussion is based largely on my experiences in leadership positions rather than on a scholarly study of leadership.

It is presumptuous of me to assume that I can reflect briefly on the "essence" of leaders and leadership. In fact, some writers assert that it is impossible to do so at all. Barnard (1948, p. 39) is one of these.

> Leaders as functioning elements of organization are not formally nominated, selected, elected or appointed, nor are they born to leadership; they are accepted and followed; and are sometimes pressed or (rarely) coerced into leading. Indeed, I have never observed any leader who was able to state adequately or intelligibly why he was able to be a leader, nor any statement of followers that acceptably expressed why they followed.

Most writers appear to agree with Barnard's assertion that leaders are not born to leadership. Obviously, however, they start with some appropriate level of intelligence, self-confidence, goal-oriented ambition, and personal attractiveness

---

*Dr. Spriestersbach is vice president for Educational Development and Research, dean of the Graduate College, and professor of Speech Pathology, University of Iowa. He is past president of the American Speech-Language-Hearing Association.

that fits given circumstances. Beyond these necessary characteristics, leadership skills can then be identified and improved upon through analysis and critique.

Although the inventory of desirable characteristics of leaders is almost endless, Barnard's list (1948) is relatively parsimonious. Indeed, the qualities he lists in order of importance are vitality and endurance, decisiveness, persuasiveness, responsibility, and intellectual capacity. Obviously he believes, and I concur, that there is a positive but relatively low correlation between intelligence and leadership capacity. Goble's list (1972, p. 96), compiled from A. H. Maslow's writings on self-actualization, is more inclusive: purposeful, realistic, creative, humble, considerate, ethical, spontaneous, self-disciplined, self-confident, and integrated. In any event, leaders and aspiring leaders would do well, from time to time, to find some means of listing their personal characteristics against some acceptable norms, so that they become aware of their strengths and weaknesses and resolve to modify the latter.

But leaders do not exist in a human vacuum. As Welsh notes (1979, p. 19): "Wherever there is human organization for the purpose of goal achievement, there are leaders." He goes on to say:

> What determines who will emerge in leadership roles, and/or how effectively leaders will perform, depends very much on the nature of the group within which they are operating, as well as on the specific features of the situation in which they must act. (p. 21)

This brings up the matter of leadership style. Likert (1961) describes four styles: exploitive-authoritative, benevolent-authoritative, consultative, and maximum participatory problem solving. Most leaders probably use some of each depending on the circumstances. However, in environments which emphasize learning and behavioral change it seems clear that leadership based on competence and the persuasiveness of ideas will be the most prosperous.

Regardless of style most authors agree on one important characteristic of leaders: a decisive sense of direction. Brown (1979, p. 54) puts it well:

> Whatever the style, a sense of direction is crucial. It is a universal requirement for leadership. The leader's sense of direction grows from imagining future possibilities, grounding plans in historical reality, and applying a consistent set of . . . convictions.

Basic to what I have said so far, and to any discussion or inquiry regarding the essence of a good leader, lies a fundamental question: How does a leader gain the consent of those being led, and hence the necessary authority to lead effectively? Fiedler and Chemers (1974) write:

> Authority does not . . . flow from the top down. A person does not have authority simply because somebody "gives" it to him. He has authority because he is accepted by his subordinates. (p. 17)
> A leader who does not recognize that his authority flows from the consent of subordinates is doomed to an unhappy if not short-lived leadership experience. (p. 10)

It takes no great insight to perceive that communication, in whatever form, is the prime vehicle at the leader's disposal for achieving consensus and concerted action from those being led. The communication must not only be clear and persuasive but must be presented in a positive and enthusiastic manner.

SOME PRAGMATIC SUGGESTIONS

At the beginning of this discussion I emphasized the necessarily personalized basis for my comments. The do's and don'ts that follow stem from my experiences. The validity of some is attested to by their inclusion in the discussion of other writers.

1. Dream the dream! Some authors talk about aiming high. I am not speaking here of silly, unrealistic dreams. Rather I mean to take due account of current realities but not to allow them to control thinking about what might be. That requires one to be clear about her or his goals and puts today's actions and problems in perspective.

2. While you are dreaming the dream think globally. It is so very easy to get bogged down with specific details before their place in the blueprint is clear. To be sure, it is easier for people to consider specifics than to think about more abstract concepts. In any event, nitpicking sometimes has a place but rarely during times when goals and directions are being developed.

3. Remember that the journey of a thousand miles begins with the first step. Important possible actions are too often talked to death. Time must be allowed, of course, for the full review of an issue, but at some point leaders must say it is time to act, even though the information available to them is incomplete and the consequences of acting are uncertain. Good leaders are willing to take reasonable risks. They do so because they have faith in their ideas and are confident that sooner or later the validity of those ideas will be recognized by colleagues within the system.

4. Believe enough in your cause that you set the highest standards for it. It is far better to be relieved as a leader because you cared too much than because you cared too little. If you adopt the highest standards, it will help you when you are faced with tough decisions.

5. Assume, until you have reason to believe otherwise, that the persons you are working with deserve your respect and appreciation for what they do, and show it. It is a rare person, regardless of his or her status, who does not appreciate appropriate stroking. And a stroke is far more apt to result in a well-motivated response than is a sneer. However, worse than a sneer is an insincere stroke. Stroking because that is what good leaders do is not enough. Strokes must be deserved and when they are, you must truly feel proud, appreciative, impressed.

6. Set a good example. Effective leaders inspire those being led. They do it by conveying an appealing vision of a better future; they do it through principled and courageous actions; they do it by demonstrating their competence. A mark of a good leader is that she or he motivates others to achieve their full potential as professionals and as human beings. A good leader unlocks the aspirations of others, and encourages the expressions of their needs, concerns and hopes through constructive actions. It follows that individuals within

organizations typically take measure of themselves by comparisons with their leaders.

7. Be absolutely trustworthy. The admonition may seem unnecessary but a great many would-be leaders do not abide by it. A successful leader's word must be her or his bond. Respect comes from the accumulation of many decisions and actions. It is difficult to erase broken words and lies from the tape.

8. Be accessible. That does not mean that you will be required to be involved in the details of your operation. Furthermore, it is not difficult to give signals about the level of involvement you intend for yourself. But being available to see your colleagues says that you are interested and that you care.

9. Communicate systematically your thinking about the goals for the organization. It can be done formally or informally, through staff meetings, briefings or memos. Any group will be more motivated to achieve a common goal if they are "in the know" and feel included in the planning and implementations designed to achieve an objective.

10. Be a good listener. Leaders do more listening than talking. They appreciate the desirability of giving others a chance to express themselves on an issue. Primarily, of course, leaders need to learn from others in considering alternative solutions for problems. Allowing others to express their views also gives them the necessary feeling of involvement. Leaders must also learn to recognize when a constructive discussion has ended. That occurs when those present have had their say, redundancy of ideas starts to appear and it becomes clear that no new information will surface at that time. The leader then ends the discussion, frequently summarizing what has been said and announcing what the next steps will be in pursuit of the matter.

11. Delegate. Most staffs enjoy, and demand, responsibility. But in delegating the leader must also make clear what the objective is for the work delegated, and what the acceptable parameters are for achieving it. Naturally the staff must proceed with the delegated responsibilities in the knowledge that they have your unqualified support, and that you will not take pleasure in "second guessing" them should they fail, as they will from time to time.

12. Recruit the brightest and the best to your organization. Very likely they will be smarter than you and almost certainly they will perform better than you in their areas of expertise. Too often people at the top are threatened by such folks. Effective leaders are not.

13. Support the advancement of your staff. Talented, well-motivated people have the ambition to advance in their fields. As a leader you must accept and support that ambition. It means that you look regularly for opportunities for them to grow professionally. It also means, of course, that you will lose some of the talented people that you have successfully recruited, and that you will be constantly bringing new, less experienced persons into your organization. The dividends for doing so are that the process creates high morale and a dynamic state of affairs so necessary for effective organizations.

14. Be accountable for your work as well as that of your staff. In your case you must be accountable to your staff as well as to your superiors. In the case of your staff you must have a regular means of keeping in touch with what they do and the results of their efforts. It is part of your responsibility to offer constructive criticism and advice when their efforts can be improved or the direction of their efforts needs to be modified.

15. Insist that your staff functions as a staff. A good staff does more than dump

problems in your lap. It also offers solutions to problems. Having agreed with your staff on the desired solutions, expect them to follow through.

16. Be a good staff person yourself! Accept the fact that you will be judged by standards higher than those of your staff. The difference in standards goes with the leader's territory.

17. Look ahead and do your homework. Be well prepared to deal with situations and do not assume that you are above rehearsing for events when necessary. Running a tight ship during meetings, saying what needs to be said within the available time, and insuring that others are appropriately involved in discussions—these things do not just happen. It is a proper and reasonable expectation of leaders that they give evidence of their preparation through their performance.

18. Respect the opinions of others and strive to demonstrate that respect on a daily basis. You do not have to like the person as a person to respect her or his opinion. Fighting about issues is easier when the combatants demonstrate respect for each other's points of view.

19. Adopt as "winning" a personal style as possible. Playing "hardnosed" may win some battles but the war is more important than the battles. In fact, the war is sometimes won with an olive branch instead of a battering ram.

20. Find ways to remain at the "state-of-the-art" level in your knowledge of the enterprise and in your enthusiasm for it. Among the ways to do this are exchanges with counterparts at conferences and seminars; identifying counterparts as role models; seeking reviews from within and without the organization of the effectiveness of your leadership, and identifying areas of your leadership which call for improvement; and taking blocks of time to be reflective about the state of your enterprise: Where are you going, where should you be going, and why? What principles are you using to get there? In what ways are your efforts enhancing or impeding the vitality of the enterprise?

21. Keep in mind that high levels of vitality and endurance are among the most commonly cited characteristics of effective leadership. You can take maximum advantage of your vitality and endurance by rejecting too many responsibilities and maintaining a strong sense of priorities in the use of your time. Without that sense you can not only fritter away your time but reduce the levels of your vitality and endurance. However, in the final analysis those levels cannot be positively manipulated unless you continue to be enthusiastic about the importance of what you are doing.

Barnard and others suggest that leadership skills are not readily transferable; rather, that they are situation-specific. It is unlikely, for example, that a national organization of physicists would be led by a sociologist. But as the purposes of organizations become more general and all-encompassing, opportunities for shifting from one leadership role to another increase. Furthermore, the capacity to shift to another role is increased if there is an unmistakable perception among your peers and associates that you are an effective leader. Certainly it is reasonable that leaders have available to them the possibilities of moving to new circumstances as part of their professional growth. So if you will take the time to be reflective about the process that has made you a leader, you can look forward to the satisfaction that comes from being tested in more than one professional arena.

Being a successful leader in any context brings with it great satisfactions, because it means you have passed a most stringent test. You have revealed what you have to offer to your colleagues and they have replied, in effect: "We like what you say and do, and we are therefore willing to join with you in our common effort. Lead us!"

REFERENCES

BARNARD, C. I. (1948). *Organization and management*. Cambridge: Harvard University Press.

BROWN, D. G. (1979). *Leadership vitality*. Washington: American Council on Education.

FIEDLER, F. E., AND M. M. CHEMERS. (1974). *Leadership and effective management*. Glenview, Ill.: Scott, Foresman and Co.

GOBLE, F. (1972). *Excellence in leadership*. Washington, D.C.: American Management Association.

LIKERT, R. (1961). *New patterns of management*. New York: McGraw-Hill.

SWANSON, S. (1984, November 29). "Leading question: What kind of people do others follow?" *Chicago Tribune*, Section 2, p. 1.

WELSH, W. A. (1979). *Leaders and elites*. New York: Holt, Rinehart and Winston.

4 Administration of Speech-Language-Hearing Programs within the University Setting

Edward J. Hardick*

Herbert J. Oyer†

INTRODUCTION

Speech, language, and hearing programs in higher education are to be found in several different settings. Latest figures show that 45 percent of the programs are in colleges of arts and sciences (including liberal arts); 22 percent in colleges of education; and 16 percent in colleges of health and/or medicine (Council of Graduate Programs in Communication Sciences and Disorders, 1984).

The larger environment in which the program is set may have a significant influence on its ability to develop in both its educational and training functions. If the unit must compete for funds with many other units within the college, the competition may be quite keen. If, however, the administrator of the speech-language and hearing unit is within a smaller college setting the program may have greater visibility and thus be more competitive for support. In either instance, however, it is the total amount of funds available to a college and the success with which the speech-language and hearing administrator interprets the needs of the organization to a dean or director that will affect the eventual outcomes of negotiations for financial support.

---

*Dr. Hardick is director of the Speech-Language-Hearing Clinic at the Ohio State University.

†Dr. Oyer is director of the Speech and Hearing Science Section, Department of Communication, at the Ohio State University.

Over the past twenty-five years there has been a substantial development of autonomy for speech-language and hearing units in colleges and universities. In the early stages of development those academic units interested in studying speech and hearing processes and the disorders that affected them were located largely in departments of speech and sometimes in psychology. Today many are set up as departments with their chairpersons or heads reporting directly to a dean. The advantages of departmental status are numerous, and include the opportunity to communicate the departmental needs directly to the college administrator who is responsible for providing financial support, greater visibility within the college and the university, and the ability to determine a course of action and direction on many issues without first securing departmental approvals.

The remainder of this chapter will discuss the responsibilities of the administrator in charge of a speech-language and hearing unit, followed by the special considerations necessary in the operation of a speech and hearing clinic.

ADMINISTRATIVE RESPONSIBILITIES

The responsibilities that rest on the shoulders of the administrator are many. They are best executed if the administrator is eminently fair in handling the many issues that surround those responsibilities, after receiving the necessary inputs from faculty and staff.

Personnel

Probably the most important responsibility concerns faculty and staff personnel: recruiting, hiring, development, periodic evaluation, recommending for promotion and/or tenure, and, when necessary, dismissing. Regardless of the many other dimensions to be considered, programs are only as strong as the personnel responsible for them. It is important in faculty recruitment that at all times a critical mass is maintained in order that all of the areas of speech-language and hearing are covered competently. An imbalance in faculty interests is ultimately reflected in curriculum and in the students' training. Fortunately, the accreditation of programs by the Educational Standards Board of the Board of Examiners of the American Speech-Language-Hearing Association helps to ensure proper balance of content within education and training programs.

The matter of promotion and tenure is of great concern to the administrator, for it has significant bearing not only upon the present status of the department, but also upon its future status. Criteria for promotion and tenure vary substantially among institutions; however, adequacy of teaching and published research are among the most frequent criteria employed.

Equal opportunity legislation has brought with it a heightened awareness of the importance of considering both gender and ethnicity when attempting to recruit faculty and staff personnel.

Students

As with faculty and staff, so it is that a program can be no stronger than the students who are studying within it. In some academic settings the chairperson of the speech-language and hearing program has little if anything to say as to the academic achievements and potentials of the undergraduate students. In other settings, however, there is the opportunity given to the chairperson to exercise discretion in the admission of undergraduates.

It is at the professional level of education and training, the masters level and at the doctoral level, that the selection of students is passed on by the graduate admissions committee and the chairperson. The chairperson's responsibility is to see to it that there is a systematic, careful, and timely processing of graduate student applications, both in fairness to the applicant and in the best interests of the program. Accredited programs must take precautions not to exceed the 6-to-1 ratio of masters students to full-time faculty for fear of jeopardizing ESB accreditation. Once admitted and matriculated, there is continuing responsibility on the part of the chairperson to assure that the student makes the best possible progress toward the degree. The astute administrator will provide for appropriate input from students and alumni for purposes of improving the program. There is no better combination for assuring the quality of a program than capable and committed students interacting with competent and caring faculty and staff.

Curriculum

The administrator is ultimately responsible for keeping the curriculum up-to-date, and is assisted tremendously by a concerned and knowledgeable curriculum committee. Once again the matter of relevant curricular offerings is brought sharply into focus by the Education and Standards Board of the American Speech-Language-Hearing Association accreditation process. The curriculum, if it is to serve well the needs of students, should not be static but rather, dynamic and ever-developing. Student appraisals and inputs into curriculum matters are important with reference to both substance and structure. A finely tuned, well-balanced, and relevant curriculum calls for an almost continuous process of evaluation. The administrator is responsible for seeing that this occurs.

Budget

The extent to which the speech-language and hearing administrator is concerned with budget will depend on the relative autonomy of the unit. If the unit is an area or section within a department, the administrator may not be responsible for any of the budget, or perhaps only for a part of it. On the other hand, if speech-language and hearing is a department, then the management of the entire budget is the administrator's concern.

Although budgets are developed somewhat differently from institution to institution, there are some common categories they share: faculty salaries, support staff salaries, supplies and services, and equipment. There may be, of course, several other accounts to be managed, to include income produced by the clinic, gifts and grants, and money paid by charitable organizations for services rendered.

The prudent administrator will exercise care in the management of the budget, with an eye toward expenditure of funds that are vital to the basic needs of the department and to assuring quality of service.

Speech-Language-Hearing Clinic

The department administrator is responsible for seeing that a training program is made available to students who are seeking clinical training and certification. In some institutions the department chairperson will also carry the title of *clinic director*; in others, however, the chairperson will appoint a faculty member as the director of the clinic. An extensive discussion of the clinic and its management appears later on in this chapter.

Facilities and Equipment

The housing provided to speech-language and hearing programs by universities varies markedly. In some instances they are located in buildings along with other departments or services, whereas in others they are located in buildings solely dedicated to the department. Whatever the location, the facility should have an adequate research laboratory and clinical training space.

If a program is to contribute to the development of new knowledge it must provide state-of-the-art equipment to the personnel engaged in research. This is costly and calls for careful planning. It is fortunate when some of the expense for equipment can be borne by grants and contracts.

Interpretation of Program Accomplishments and Needs

It is highly important that the department chairperson communicates the achievements and needs of the faculty and students to those relevant administrators within the university. Opportunity for this occurs in a formal way through annual reports or other special reports. The informal communication of accomplishments and needs can also be effective.

Communicating the clinical objectives of the program to groups outside the university is also important, as it can attract potential clients to the clinic and financial support from charitable organizations.

Scheduling of Faculty and Staff Loads

Several criteria must be employed as the chairperson of the department sets about scheduling the responsibilities of faculty and staff. The most important is that of competency in a particular area. Another is interest on the part of faculty and staff in being involved with certain responsibilities. A third is the need for certain responsibilities to be covered for the sake of completeness of program. It is critical that the administrator make assignments in the best interests of students, faculty, and staff. It is also very important that loads are distributed in such a manner that all are carrying their fair share of the work of the department.

Interprofessional Relationships

Because of the multidimensionality of the study of speech-language and hearing and the disorders thereof, it is necessary for relationships to be established with other professionals in the university and the larger community. These often serve as sources of referral to the clinical training program as well as sources to whom referrals may be made. The establishing of these lines of relationship need not be made solely by the administrator but by faculty and staff as well. It is the responsibility of the administrator, however, to see that they are made.

Service Courses

Within any academic setting the speech-language and hearing program is quite costly as compared with other programs that attract large numbers of students. The administrator is wise who seeks to make available the contents of speech-language and hearing by way of service courses to students preparing to be, for example, teachers, child development specialists, nurses, gerontologists, occupational therapists, or physical therapists. Not only does this pass basic information along to future professionals of other disciplines, but it also reduces the cost of instruction.

Faculty and Staff Meetings

It is highly important that faculty and staff have the opportunity to meet periodically to evaluate the work of the department, to deal with special problems, and to engage in planning for the future. Although such meetings provide the opportunity for the administrator to pass along information that is important to the total enterprise and that would not normally reach the faculty/staff, they should not be used simply for a sustained monologue by the administrator.

Faculty and staff meetings provide the ideal setting for systematic reporting of committees at work on special concerns such as curriculum, graduate admissions, equipment, and laboratory management. The frequency of these meetings is dependent upon the needs of each department. They should be held frequently enough so that faculty/staff don't lose their sense of continuity and unity of purpose.

Research

Still another responsibility of the administrator is to encourage systematic programs of research. Efforts at research not only develop new knowledge, but in doing so they help to make teaching and learning a more exciting process. This can have a stimulating effect on students, who then try to develop their own research or to extend a professor's research.

Both the public and private sectors have been very helpful through the years in supporting research in communicative disorders. If the administrator expects research productivity from faculty, the teaching load, available equipment, suitable laboratory facilities and support must all be considered. Encouraging the faculty to develop and submit proposals to granting agencies is also important.

Morale

There are many variables that can affect the morale of a group. High morale on the part of faculty, staff, and students is an important ingredient of a successful program. Although it in no way assures maximum productivity, high morale makes the many tasks to be accomplished somewhat easier. The administrator is the key to the development and maintenance of high morale. A sense of trust in the administrator who listens carefully, who is sensitive and completely fair in the handling of issues and problems, and who shows genuine care for personnel, students, and the program, is of paramount importance. Additionally, the less complex the formal structure of the department the greater the chance for individual expression of attitudes and thus the greater the feeling of integration. It is this sense of integration as opposed to alienation that improves the quality of human relationships and ultimately group morale.

CLINIC ADMINISTRATION

Educational programs in speech-language and hearing in American colleges and universities maintain some form of clinical service program as the basic site for the professional preparation of speech-language pathologists and audiologists. These clinics have much in common with other speech and hearing clinics in organizational structures quite different from those within the university. They all provide services to a range of disorders and ages, engage in public education, and have problems in funding, personnel, and interprofessional and agency relationships. They all strive to deliver high-quality service in the most meaningful and expedient manner, are concerned with quality control of services, and sincerely attempt to meet the highest standards of ethical practice in the treatment of patients. There are areas of administration, therefore, that are common to clinical programs in diverse settings. Much that is presented in other parts of this book will apply equally well to a clinical facility associated with a university's educational program. There are some differences, however, that are unique to those clinics engaging in education and the training of professionals in speech-language and hearing. Emphasis here will be given to those areas and issues that are unique to the university setting.

General Description of the Speech and Hearing Clinic
in a University Setting

Our concern is with those academic units known by such names as the Department of Communicative Disorders, Audiology and Speech Sciences, Speech-language Pathology and Audiology, and Speech and Hearing Science. Their primary mission is to prepare speech and hearing professionals. Not included are those clinics, usually in medical schools, which do not have as their primary function the clinical training of speech and hearing students. University clinics associated with academic units exist primarily to serve a professional education purpose as a laboratory for clinical training of students working toward certification and licensure as speech-language pathologists and audiologists. They also serve as research laboratories where data about the clinical and training processes are collected. In other words, their function as a training and research center is the fundamental reason for their existence. However, it is imperative to understand that this in no way subordinates patient welfare to training and research goals. It is the balance between these important purposes that gives the university clinic its unique character.

Because its primary mission is the educational preparation of professionals, the organization of a university training clinic is unique to that setting and purpose. The mission of the clinic within the larger structure of the university provides an orientation towards clinic dynamics, that is, faculty participation, scheduling, use of time, fee structure, and relationship of patients to staff, which is sufficiently different to warrant consideration apart from other clinical service programs.

University clinics are operated as integral components of the department providing the educational program. How they are administered, and the make-up of the staff, varies from one institution to another. Some clinics are operated as somewhat self-supporting enterprises while others are totally funded by the educational budget of the department; some are accredited, others not. Given that the university clinic and its host department may be located in various colleges, and that a particular college may imprint certain characteristics on the clinic, in general the clinics are fairly similar as a result of external factors such as requirements of clinical certification, licensure, and accreditation.

Thus far we have talked only of clinics that are an outgrowth of the educational program operated and controlled by the university faculty. One variation of this structure is sufficiently different to warrant mention. In some communities a linking together of a service agency and a university program has occurred through mutual agreement whereby the agency provides a facility and basic clinical staff, and the university provides land or some other inducement that makes a joint venture attractive to both parties. The resulting facility houses a clinical program responsible to a board of trustees or directors independent of the university and the academic or research program of the department which is responsible to university administration. There may be separate budgets, but in most other respects the programs function under a common set of rules, including personnel selection. This form of organization is, nevertheless, more complicated than the simple model of most university clinics. With two governing or controlling bodies the potential for conflict increases. However, there are several university-community clinic organizational structures around the country that have achieved considerable success in education, clinical programming, and research.

Professional Staff

The professional staff of a university clinic is frequently made up of the faculty, some full or part-time master's level clinical supervisors, and perhaps clinically certified graduate students holding part-time appointments. The faculty are employed by the university to teach and conduct research. Their salaries derive from the university budget and are unaffected by the clinic's financial balance. Promotion, tenure, and salary increases for faculty are based on the number of students taught, the quality of instruction, and the quantity and quality of research productivity. The amount of time spent in clinical activities serving patient needs and supervising student trainees is not a significant variable in comparison to teaching large classes, generating research funds, and publishing. As a result many faculty members choose to minimize the amount of time they devote to clinical practice or supervising student trainees, and display little interest in the business affairs of the clinic. Of course, this situation does not exist at all institutions, as some value teaching and service more highly; others stress research, teaching, and service, in that order. In any case, faculty can be considered only as part-time clinical staff because they do have other responsibilities—in the classroom, advising, in committee service, and in direction of student research. Be that as it may, many faculty members do participate in clinical activities directly or as supervisors because they view it as essential for good teaching and as a means of conducting applied research or as a means of generating research ideas. Some departments have evolved satisfactory criteria for clinical involvement of faculty members as part of their teaching or research loads; however, there is always the possibility of changes in university criteria with new administrative leadership or as severe economic threats force review of faculty roles. Therefore, the involvement of faculty in the activities of the clinic is a perennial problem, more or less severe depending on the goals and values of the institution. As a result those departments having doctoral programs often rely on doctoral students holding appropriate clinical certification to devote one-quarter to one-half of their time to clinical supervision. While there is merit in this assignment, because teaching experience is gained, it can be detrimental to the student if such assignments interfere with learning experiences in research laboratories, for example; and it can be detrimental to the program when inconsistencies in the range and quality of services arise over time due to variations in students' clinical interests and the transient nature of their appointments. Often they are pressed into service without due regard for program needs, and often they do not have the experience necessary to take a leadership role in supervision of student trainees. For many reasons reliance on these appointments as the major means of supervision and clinical training is questionable.

A survey of university clinics would reveal the variations in staffing supervision just discussed. Some programs rely upon regular faculty members to provide all supervision, some rely on a combination of faculty members and doctoral students, while some rely on full-time supervisors with varying degrees of assistance from faculty and doctoral students.

Fees for Service

For the most part speech-language and hearing clinics in university settings in the past did not charge fees for services. A major reason was that employment was limited to public schools or to military and VA hospitals where direct fees for service were nonexistent. Training programs were viewed within that same model. Clinical expenses were minimal in this fledgling field; there were few published and standardized tests and materials, and hearing-testing equipment was limited to an audiometer and a phonograph. The costs of clinical operation were borne by the academic unit as a necessary educational expense associated with the teaching and research programs. Fee schedules were eventually introduced as the field matured and technology developed. Since then there has been an explosive increase in the number of commercial tests and materials available. There has also been an increase in sophisticated audiometric equipment as research into hearing disorders has led to new tests and the development of instrumentation to evaluate the auditory system. In addition there has been an increase in requests for professionals by institutions outside the educational and military settings. Thus has the model been revised. Speech-language and hearing clinics increasingly requested administrative approval for an income-producing account and a fee schedule. Progress was slow because the profession, and the public, had become accustomed to free services. In fact there are still some college and university clinics that provide free services.

The nature of the fees account and uses that can be made of the income are determined by the university. In some cases, clinic income is deposited into the university's general fund, in other cases the funds remain in the fees account and can be expended by the department within specified limits. These accounts are audited by the university to ensure adherence to commonly accepted bookkeeping procedures and the legitimacy of expenditures. The profession has matured to the point that speech-language pathologists and audiologists, in general, are aware that they have valuable services to render, that there is a cost involved, and that these services should be paid for by the patient or a third party. However, there are still clinicians who are uncomfortable discussing fees with patients and are prone to waive fees for the slightest of reasons. Fees charged by university clinics are usually less than in other clinics in the community, not unlike the practice of other clinical disciplines providing services in the university. This is understandable because much of the work is done by students-in-training, who tend to proceed more slowly than experienced practitioners. The fee schedule has to be reviewed periodically in order to keep abreast of contemporary trends and in light of the financial needs of the clinic.

Today, more than ever, a university clinic is run much as any business enterprise requiring the managerial skills of an administrator to develop the annual budget and to review and analyze income and expense statements. The growth of the university clinic as a revenue-producing unit has been reinforced of late as university administrators, in their quest for adequate economic support, have turned to income-producing accounts as a source of assistance. Thus we find the imposition of a percentage overhead charge on monthly income (5.5 percent at our institution) that goes to the general fund. Reviews of financial statements for income/expenditure balances, and adjustments in the fee schedule, are necessary for planning acquisitions of new technical instruments and for replacing lost, damaged, or obsolete equipment and materials.

Administrative Models

An issue of some concern is how the speech-language and hearing clinic is to be administered. Should the chairperson of the department also serve as director of the clinic? Should some other faculty member serve as director and chief administrator of the clinic, responsible to the chairperson of the department? Should the director of the clinic be someone other than a faculty member? Should the several components of the clinic, that is, hearing clinic, speech clinic, and language clinic, be operated separately by their respective staffs? Examples of these models can be found in university clinics today. The model utilized in a particular program will be influenced by local factors including the interpersonal dynamics of the people involved, and whether the components are housed in the same facility or must be operated at different locations. These are questions that must be answered in each locality taking into account physical and personal factors.

Administrative Responsibilities
in University Clinic Management

Sensitivity to others and effective communication are critical elements for smooth operation of a clinical service given the multiple needs of staff, students, and patients. The first goal of any university clinic is the delivery of quality care to the patients. A secondary goal is the development of an organizational structure that produces an environment conducive to efficient operation and learning. There has to be a chain of command and levels of authority, but every effort must be made to avoid abuse of one's position and arrogant pursuit of individual interests to the exclusion of the common good. Roles and responsibilities must be specified for all levels within the clinic as the first step towards a comfortable but productive work environment. Good working relationships are facilitated by an organizational structure planned and developed by students, staff, and faculty.

There are five major areas of administrative responsibility in clinics in which the primary function is the training of practitioners: personnel management, financial management, scheduling, accreditation, and supervision.

Personnel management. The staff of a university speech-language and hearing clinic consists of four types of personnel: students engaging in clinical practice toward completion of clinical certification requirements; teaching associates who, while enrolled as graduate students, are paid as part-time clinical supervisors; clinical supervisors, employed part- or full-time as permanent staff; and the faculty.

Effective management of a heterogeneous group requires a structure sufficiently defined for individuals to know their responsibilities and limitations. Certain administrative principles seem evident if the university clinic program is to achieve optimum success. A basic principle concerns enumeration of the responsibilities and powers of the professional clinical staff, including the director. Positive relationships and a smoothly operating organization are enhanced by a set of clearly written guidelines setting forth the duties and responsibilities of the individuals at each organizational level. The director plays a major role in creating a desirable environment in the workplace (Keys, 1964). It is therefore essential that the responsibilities and authority of the clinic director be agreed upon perhaps in the form of a position description made available to other members of the staff, and that the director adhere to its provisions.

Next, the administrative structure of the clinic should be clearly defined and its relationship to the academic and research programs of the department specified. This administrative structure determines how the clinic will be run and begins to clarify duties and responsibilities that might be delegated, and to whom they are assigned. The reason it is necessary to delineate the relationship between the clinic director and the department is to facilitate the harmonious interaction of the teaching and research faculty with the ongoing clinical program. If a clinic is to prosper it is imperative that the director have complete knowledge of the activities of all involved and be aware of the demands placed on staff, students, and patients. To permit individual faculty members without review or approval to collect data or institute new clinical procedures is antithetical to efficient operation and may be hazardous to staff morale and public relations.

The wise clinical director will not retain all authority, because this is inefficient and not conducive to fostering the sense of involvement, trust, and leadership development that characterize a desirable work environment. In a university clinic there are many responsibilities to be assigned. Whether they are assigned to the director or the clinical staff must be decided by the people involved. There are, however, certain responsibilities that probably should be retained by the director. Matters pertaining to financial affairs including the fee schedule, authority to waive fees, and control over the operating budget; issues pertaining to salary; and cost accounting. Such matters as public relations, facilities, financial support, personnel issues, employment practices, and faculty requests for clinical or research involvement should also be the responsibility of the director. Other responsibilities which can be delegated to the supervisory staff include those pertaining to equipment needs; maintenance; calibration; materials; the development of new programs; intake and discharge criteria; scheduling and assignment of student trainees; methods of evaluating student and supervisory staff performance; a code of conduct and clinical protocols for student clinicans; and development of quality-assurance procedures. All recommendations derived from delegated responsibilities should be discussed, modified, and approved by the whole staff or by a representative executive committee. Once duties have been delegated, the wise administrator will not intervene unsolicited; this often destroys enthusiasm and motivation. All policy decisions should be in writing and shared with the staff and placed in appropriate clinical manuals. Needless to say they should be reviewed periodically and revised as necessary.

Financial management.   Although there are many similarities in the financial management of speech-language and hearing clinics in the various settings, there are sufficient differences to warrant separate discussion of the university clinics that are components of graduate educational programs.

The clinics not deriving income from patient fees receive funding from the university to cover most costs. Additional funds are sometimes obtained through grants and gifts. Departmental (including clinic) budgets are obtained through budget hearings between the administrator and higher level administrators. Proposed budgets compete with those of other departments and the funds granted are limited by the ability of the university to secure sufficient funding from its sources, that is, the legislature, tuition, grants, and gifts. The funds requested cover, for example, personnel, equipment and maintenance, materials, consumable supplies, travel, and communications. Once the funds have been obtained, financial management consists of allocating them as projected, and monitoring expenditures so that at the end of the fiscal year all monies have been expended, the allocation has not been exceeded, and most of the projected needs have been met. The process is then repeated for the next fiscal year.

The majority of clinics charge fees for services and the income is deposited in the clinic account maintained by the university business office. The clinic account does not replace departmental accounts for salaries, equipment, and the operating expenses of a teaching-research program. The clinic account differs from the depart mental accounts in that deposits can be accepted from outside sources, that is, clinic fees are paid. These are referred to as *rotary* accounts because monies can be deposited as well as expended. The university's business office provides a detailed monthly statement of income and expenditure. Some universities permit a cash balance to be carried over from one year to the next even though the clinical operation, as part of the university organization, is expected to be nonprofit. Carryover of funds is necessary to accumulate financial reserves for replacing expensive equipment. The ideal situation exists when there are not personnel or overhead (rent or utilities) expenses encumbering the clinic account; the assumption being that it is the university's responsibility to provide teaching and support personnel, facilities, and basic equipment for educational programs. Often, however, administrative philosophy or economic pressures require the university clinic account to support some personnel costs as well as contribute to overhead expenses. Expenditures from the clinic income account are generally applied to such items as personnel, equipment, supplies and services, communications, printing and reproduction, student wages and tuition, travel, fees (audit collection and legal), accreditation, advertising, staff recruitment, dues and licenses, staff training, and continuing education.

There must be sufficient income before funds can be committed; deficit spending is not permitted, so careful management and planning are necessary. The determination of fees is based upon at least three related factors: reasonable and customary fees charged by other clinical programs in the region; the number of potential patients; and the income required to meet basic budget needs. Financial management of a university clinic is, therefore, a dynamic process requiring frequent review and revision. Long-range planning is required to replace or purchase new equipment and, if personnel are included, future salary and fringe benefit increases must be provided for. Attention is required to assure the necessary caseload, otherwise income will be reduced and the budget jeopardized. Fee increases must be carefully considered so that they do not reduce the patient population and imperil clinic operation. Another matter requiring administrative attention is whether or not the university clinic should engage in dispensing products to its patients, or utilize an alternative approach with similar results for the patient.

The alternative approach alluded to is the one we have selected, and apparently it is utilized by some other university clinics. In the audiology section of the clinic, for example, our fee schedule includes charges for all services performed including evaluation, earmold impressions, fitting the aid, providing training in the use and maintenance of the hearing aid, repairs, and annual reevaluations. The product (hearing aid) is purchased directly by the patient from one of the mail-order distributors approved by a certified audiologist. The amplification system is delivered to the clinic for an electroacoustic analysis before fitting. The only hardware directly obtained is a laboratory fabricated earmold system from an impression taken by the staff. When these components have arrived the client is contacted for fitting and training. The fee charged for fitting also covers an additional visit to the clinic prior to termination of the thirty-day trial. Since the fitting fee can be in reasonable balance with the costs of hearing aids obtained in more traditional ways, we do not feel the need to dispense directly, because additional costs for record keeping and inventory maintenance are then incurred. The educational benefits of direct dispensing over this alternative fitting method are insignificant because actual costs in a university are unknown and cannot form the basis for pricing. In a university setting the real value of dispensing or fitting is in the professional management of the process.

Another aspect of financial and patient management requiring attention is that of third-party payment for services. Medicare, Medicaid, Blue Cross/Blue Shield, Vocational Rehabilitation, Crippled Children's Service, and the various insurance companies underwriting the UAW or related contracts for hearing rehabilitation services have complex and variable procedures and payment schedules. Learning what is covered, under what conditions, and the amount of reimbursement, is important so that no disservice is done to the patient or to the clinic. The many facets of financial planning and management require continuous analysis by the administrator to ensure income stability and the growth necessary to support the budget.

Accreditation. Another dimension of administration is one shared with all clinical facilities desirous of achieving the highest standards of professional performance and the assurance of quality programming to the community, related professions, and to third-party purchasers. Since Professional Services Board (PSB) accreditation of a clinical program is not unique to a university system, administrative responsibilities in the general development of procedures consistent with accreditation standards will not be discussed. However, meeting accreditation standards in a university clinic presents some additional problems because of the training nature of the program. Large numbers of students are in the clinic at any given time; the group is not static, that is, new students enter each term while others leave through graduation or other assignments. At all times the number of students exceeds that of the staff. Staff, therefore, have the difficult and continuous responsibility for supervision of students at different levels of development. They must also familiarize students with accreditation and certification requirements, in addition to the purely professional issues involved in disorder intervention. This means that the professional staff, in addition to developing policies and procedures consistent with current accreditation standards, must develop mechanisms for student awareness so that the program can function smoothly at the highest level of professional performance and maintain adequate records for validation.

The supervisory process.   The major responsibility of the clinical staff in a training program is to provide sensitive supervision of student clinicians in an environment supportive to the professional development of each individual; and, at the same time, to provide an exemplary model to motivate the student toward clinical excellence. The administration of the supervisory dimension of clinical practice is characterized by four aspects, each of which has a strong influence on the atmosphere of the training program, the adequacy of the clinician at graduation, and the quality of service to patients. These aspects are choice of supervisory personnel; patient-clinician scheduling; the dynamics of supervision; and the evaluation of student performance.

Supervisory personnel.   Increasing attention has been directed toward the preparation of trained clinical supervisors and the identification of desirable characteristics of supervisors and the supervisory process. Research in supervision and the teaching of this content are legitimate components of the educational process (Dowling, 1979; Culatta and Helmick, 1981; Anderson, 1981). Historically, the amount and quality of supervision has been very uneven, resulting in weakness in the preparation of clinicians. Identifying optimal personal characteristics of supervisors, refining methods of interacting with student clinicians, and standardizing the supervisory process have been worthwhile developments. It is now possible for clinical administrators to interview prospective supervisors with a set of criteria. The expanding literature on the subject also makes it feasible for university clinics to offer inservice training for staff supervisors, including faculty members who participate in supervision. The administrator of a university speech and hearing clinic should provide encouragement and support for staff participation in workshops, courses, or less formal activities designed to improve the supervisory process and individual skills.

Clinician-patient scheduling.   A recurring responsibility of a university clinic staff is the assignment of student clinicians to patients. This task occurs at the beginning of every school term and is a time-consuming and frustrating process. Given the necessity of providing each student with experiences in diagnosis and therapy, with children and adults, with the various disorders of communication, and of providing experience in more than one type of setting, the complexity of the task is obvious. Current records of each student's clinical experience and academic background must be reviewed to assure that orderly progress toward certification requirements has been made, and that students have the appropriate academic background before clinical assignments are made. Supervisors must be knowledgeable of students needs and interests, patient needs, and whether or not their personal characteristics are conducive to a constructive relationship. Beyond pairing clinician and patient, the choice of supervisor for each pair must be determined. Good administration means the presence of adequate systems for maintaining current clinical and academic records and the development of policies and procedures for completing the scheduling process in an expeditious and equitable manner.

Dynamics of supervision. Accreditation of the academic program specifies minimal criteria for supervision, restricted primarily to the amount of time direct supervision must occur. Other aspects of the supervisory process, such as the nature and frequency of conferences, are left to the discretion of the staff or the individuals involved. Supervision that promotes student growth and patient welfare is the goal, and requires the thoughtful cooperation of staff and students. Interactions between supervisor and student are of a very special teaching nature involving both advising and counseling. The dynamics of the supervisory process include the number and type of conferences, elements of the evaluative process, the manner in which observation will be conducted, and the supervisor's role with the patient and family. Other matters also pertaining to the nature of the supervisor–student clinician interaction need to be formalized so that all parties know their responsibilities, deadlines, and methods of appeal. It is the responsibility of the administrator to see that attention is given to these matters and that the policies and procedures are disseminated. Supervisors in outside sites should participate, if possible, in any deliberations, or at least be thoroughly briefed to provide a consistent set of expectations for students in all facilities associated with the training program. Fortunately, ASHA committees have been discussing the supervisory process and have made important recommendations in the areas mentioned (Committee on Supervision and Council on Professional Standards, 1982; Committee on Supervision, 1982; Committee on Supervision, 1984).

Evaluation of student performance. This is frequently a troublesome area because of the difficulty in identifying the critical elements in a therapeutic interaction, quantifying human behavior in a therapeutic relationship, and assessing quality of performance. Nevertheless, experienced clinicians do seem to agree in identifying the "good" and the "less-than-adequate" student clinicians. A university clinical staff may develop its own protocol for evaluating student performance. They will have to for some experiences, or they may choose to adopt widely disseminated tools such as the *Wisconsin Procedure for Appraisal of Clinical Competence* (Shriberg et al., 1975), or the audiology practicum evaluation procedure of Frank (1980). The staff must develop procedures to ensure that student clinicians receive prior information concerning the skills they are expected to develop, and the criteria by which they will be evaluated. Providing this information in advance is imperative because not all supervisors share the same expectations and priorities.

A related issue concerns inflation of grades in clinical practica. Too often they seem higher than warranted. This is unfair to superior clinicians and often compromises the counseling of others. Evaluation of grading practices should be reviewed periodically.

SUGGESTIONS TO FUTURE SPEECH-LANGUAGE AND HEARING ADMINISTRATORS IN A UNIVERSITY CLINIC

The ways in which a university speech-language and hearing clinic differs from others are related to its primary mission, education, and the setting in which it is located. It is an institution requiring more than clinical service from its staff, and given to periodic downtime in certain of its activities. The clinical components of the educational program in audiology and speech-language pathology have grown in size, number of services, population served, and quality of service. The results of clinical research, accreditation, and licensing have stimulated development of clinical service and training facilities that are the equal of any other similar disciplines. The increasing complexity of clinical operation from business and service perspectives, and from its sensitivity to human rights and needs, has developed to the point where several conclusions seem warranted.

The modern program in audiology and speech-language pathology requires a division of labor where the administrative responsibility for the clinical service program should be delegated to an appointed clinical director while the department chairperson assumes administrative responsibility for the academic unit. Indeed, an increasing number of training programs have adopted this model. The model would make the clinical director responsible to the department chairperson who would retain final authority in matters of basic policy, relationships with other components of the department, and the use of the clinic income. The need for a full-time administrator is further supported by the rapid expansion of computer technology which will significantly change not only the delivery of services but the handling of data, budget, records, and communications. The clinical director could be a full-time administrative or professional employee or a faculty member who can combine administration, teaching, and clinical research. Some programs decide that codirectors are preferable, one from each of the clinical divisions.

A second suggestion is that university clinics in departments providing professional education should charge fees for the services offered the public. However, salaries of the core staff and faculty should come from the general salary budget of the university because these people are performing functions central to the institution's educational mission. The training of speech and hearing personnel is expensive compared to that of personnel in fields outside the health-related professions. Since university funds often tend to be allocated on the basis of the number of students served, most programs would find it advantageous to have an additional source of funds independent of the university budget. In addition, it is high time we accepted that the good we do for communicatively impaired patients is worthy of compensation. Programs not charging fees are not realistic in light of the costs involved in providing quality service within the university setting. As indicated previously, salaries of the core staff and faculty should come from the general salary budget of the university because these people are performing functions central to the institution's mission: education.

A third suggestion is presented, although it has been discussed only indirectly. The faculty who teach, do research, and provide some clinical supervision should be supplemented by full-time clinical supervisors, minimally masters level, who are employed as professional rather than as academic staff, and employed on a year-round basis. On many campuses this type of employee has equal protection and fringe benefits as the faculty but is not within a tenure pattern. A probationary period usually precedes the granting of job security. This position classification is preferable to a tenure track position wherein these employees must meet the same criteria as faculty or, if not, are granted tenure by a double standard. A double standard for tenure weakens the system, while imposing faculty criteria for tenure produces an unacceptably threatening environment for staff who usually do not have the credentials for research, nor the time for scholarly activity. It is desirable for the professional staff to have year-round appointments because some basic services of the clinic should be available on a full-time basis. Patients need to be scheduled and other office work must continue; hearing aids and earmolds need to be dispensed, repaired, or modified; and laryngectomized patients may need prosthetic services. The modern university speech and hearing clinic is a full-time business.

SUMMARY

University teaching-training-research programs are complex organizations requiring talented leadership. The administrator's primary responsibility is to provide a physical and collegial environment where faculty can be productive, students can flourish in the pursuit of knowledge, and where the professional development of clinicians has an equally high priority.

Developing methods to accomplish these goals is the challenge the administrator faces. The faculty, staff, and students must be encouraged to participate in program evaluation and development, and they must be willing to assume some supportive administrative responsibilities. Developing and maintaining organized momentum in the program, keeping a balance between faculty-staff needs and students educational requirements, providing sound fiscal management while seeking ways to improve resources, and serving as an articulate advocate of the program and profession are some characteristics of the effective administrator. Modern programs in speech-language and hearing are large enough that levels of administration are required to provide necessary attention to all phases of the program. The effective administrator is willing to delegate authority, and encourages freedom for the exercise of that authority, while retaining ultimate authority for decisions.

REFERENCES

ANDERSON, JEAN L. (February 1981). "Training of supervisors in speech-language pathology and audiology," *Asha*, 23, 77–82.

COMMITTEE ON SUPERVISION, AND COUNCIL ON PROFESSIONAL STANDARDS. (May 1982). "Minimum qualifications for supervisors and suggested competencies for effective clinical supervision," *Asha*, 24, 339–342.

COMMITTEE ON SUPERVISION. (December 1982). "Suggested competencies for effective clinical supervision," *Asha*, 24, 1021–1023.

COMMITTEE ON SUPERVISION. (May 1984). "Clinical supervision in speech-language pathology and audiology," *Asha*, 26, 45–48.

COUNCIL OF GRADUATE PROGRAMS IN COMMUNICATION SCIENCES AND DISORDERS. (September 1984). *1983-84 National Survey*, P.O. Box 1903, University, Ala. 35486.

CULATTA, RICHARD A. (December 1980). "Clinical supervision: The state of the art (Part I)," *Asha*, 22, 985–993.

CULATTA, RICHARD AND JOSEPH W. HELMICK. (January 1981). "Clinical supervision: The state of the art (Part II)," *Asha*, 23, 21–31.

DOWLING, SUSANN. (September 1979). "The teaching clinic: A supervisory alternative," *Asha*, 21, 646–649.

FRANK, TOM. (April 1980). "A skill-based clinical audiology practicum evaluation procedure," *Asha*, 22, 251–254.

KEYS, JOHN W. (December 1964). "Administration," *Asha*, 6, 477–486.

5 Public School Speech-Language-Hearing Administration

Gloria L. Engnoth*

INTRODUCTION

Of the children and youth attending school, there are many who exhibit speech-language disorders or some degree of hearing impairment. In general, where speech-language disorders are defined by abnormal performance on actual tests, information suggests that between 10 and 15 percent of children ages 6-7 years, 4 and 6 percent of children age 11 years, and 1 and 2 percent of youth age 17 years have speech-language problems (Leske, 1981). In addition, data suggest that there are between 2 and 3 million school children with some degree of hearing impairment. Included in these numbers are children with middle-ear infections resulting in conductive loss; children with sensorineural hearing loss; and those with central auditory processing problems (Eagles et al., 1963; Berg and Fletcher, 1970; Ross and Giolas, 1978).

All of these children attend schools. Each requires an appropriate program of therapeutic intervention to assist him or her in coping with the effects of the handicap upon the learning process. Schools then become the most viable environment in which to provide speech-language-hearing services.

---

*Dr. Engnoth is coordinator of special education for the Baltimore County Public Schools, Maryland.

Several basic factors support the organization and administration of speech-language-hearing services as part of school programs of instruction. First, schools have an identified mission. That mission is to develop the individual's inborn capacities to the fullest extent consistent with social welfare (Moehlman, 1951). Therefore, schools arrange a broad spectrum of instructional programs and support systems to assist each student in achieving this goal. From the earliest grades on, achieving competency in oral and written communication is a primary objective of school programs. Today, in fact, many states have mandated assessment to assure basic competency in these areas. Since speech-, language-, and hearing-handicapped students are at risk in attaining oral and written language competencies, any interference with the achievement of these competencies must be eliminated or circumvented. Speech-language-hearing service is the primary support system selected to fulfill this role.

Secondly, society preconditions children and youth attitudes toward achieving an appropriate education by attending school. Children and youth know that they come to school to learn. They are aware that their parents expect them to do well in school. Further, they understand that they must learn academic skills by successfully completing work provided by their teachers.

Children and youth also understand that there are resources open to them that will assist them in achieving success. Services that support achievement of success in oral and written competency are welcomed and viewed as part of the school program. Students with communication handicaps generally, then, have few negative attitudes about receiving speech-language-hearing services. In fact, these services have become so well integrated that parents and students often express surprise and dismay when these children are classified as being handicapped.

Attitudes of school administrators and instructional personnel to the provision of assistance to students with speech-language-hearing disorders are also supportive. Any interventions that enhance students' successful performance in the classroom and reduce the teacher's obligation to provide "additional help" are indeed welcomed. If speech-language-hearing services programs are organized, administered and implemented appropriately, close working relationships between administrators, teachers, speech-language pathologists and audiologist emerge and flourish. In fact, the coordination of instruction, therapeutic intervention and monitoring activities related to student emerging competencies tend to promote positive professional interactions which facilitate student habilitation.

The third factor which supports the organization and administration of speech-language-hearing programs in schools is indeed unique. Though these services can be accessed in hospitals, community agencies, university training centers and private practice facilities, only public schools have federal and state mandates to provide them. As has been described before, schools have made speech-language services available for a long time. However, these services have not been readily available in every school district. If the community supported their inclusion, if the professional staff did not view them as intrusive upon instructional time, and if the financial support was substantial enough to permit support services, speech-language-hearing services were provided. If they were not included, it became the parents' responsibility to make private arrangements to obtain them.

In the early 1970s the emergence of the civil rights movement and legal activities on the part of parents whose severely handicapped children were not included in public education programs brought about a monumental change in the organization and administration of education and support services to handicapped children and youth.

In 1975, the ninety-fourth Congress passed the Education of All Handicapped Children Act (P.L. 94-142). In addition, in 1977 the United States Office of Education, through the Bureau of Health, Education, and Welfare produced regulations which implemented amendments to part B of the act. These regulations govern the provision of grant funds to state and local education agencies to assist them in the education of handicapped children. They also include provisions designed to: (1) assure that all handicapped children have available to them a free appropriate public education (FAPE); (2) assure that the rights of the handicapped and their parents are protected ("due process"); (3) assist states and localities in providing for the education of handicapped children; and (4) assess and assure the effectiveness of efforts to educate such children. Further, the regulations include the rules for counting and reporting handicapped children to the federal government (the All Handicapped Children Act, 1975).

Public participation in the initiation of the legislation and the development of the regulations was extensive. This high level of participation is continuing. It is demonstrated by parents being directly involved in decisions pertaining to their children's assessment, individualized educational planning and placement; by citizens providing consultation to boards of education through serving on state and local school district citizen advisory committees; and by advocacy groups and special education personnel joining in carefully analyzing, providing testimony and lobbying for or against proposed changes in regulations at the national and state governmental levels.

The implementation of the Education of All Handicapped Children Act has affected children and youth, parents, teachers, school administrators, training institutions and their programs. The intent of the legislation was not that of influencing only those segments of school systems charged with educating the handicapped, but rather the reorganization of the entire education system to provide comprehensive educational services to them (Podemski et al., 1984).

The impact of P.L. 94-142 has been substantial and beneficial. Positive philosophical and operational commitments have been demonstrated and the provision of equal opportunity for a free appropriate education has been assured for all children. The various aspects of the law and its regulations have (1) produced state law and regulations which reaffirm and reinforce the national commitment; (2) altered the role and responsibilities of state education and local school districts in providing education and related services to all children; (3) changed the organization and administration of departments charged with the responsibility of delivering services to the handicapped; and (4) affected the processes and interactions of professional staff members designated as providing services to handicapped and non-handicapped students.

In many respects the administrator of speech-language-hearing services in schools has an ideal environment in which to implement services. Not only is there an identified population which is readily accessible and positively motivated to participate, and a legal mandate for organizing and providing these services, but also federal, state and local fiscal support. In addition there is a ready-made and functioning organization which facilitates delivery of speech pathology and audiology services to students. The key to the administration of a program of speech-language-hearing services in the schools is the administrator's provision of a design which combines positive parent/teacher attitudes and appropriate clinical philosophies and techniques, and embeds them in a highly organized, structured educational system which is already in place. This is more easily written than accomplished. Perhaps the first step toward providing quality administrative practice is to understand the underlying organization and operation of educational programs.

ORGANIZATION AND ADMINISTRATION
OF PUBLIC SCHOOL SYSTEMS

"The American public school is conceived as a classless, impartial, nonpartisan, non-sectarian agency through which all children may receive instruction. It is the common meeting place for the harmonization of those cultural differences which otherwise create social conflict and group cleavage" (Moehleman, 1951). Implementation of this concept has resulted in the evolution of public education as a cooperative endeavor between the family and government.

Direct control over public education has been a function of the community and serves to protect it from use or misuse by the state and federal government. While the state has been vested with plenary powers in the issues pertaining to education by the Constitution, each community through a decentralized organization has maintained local control and thereby protected education from outside political influences.

ORGANIZATION OF PUBLIC EDUCATION

The organization of public education is described in the literature according to governmental district (for example, state, intermediate, local school district); size (for example, large school districts, medium-sized school districts, small school district); and/or location (for example, urban, suburban, rural).

The basic unit in the organization of public education is the *local unit*, the school district. It is a quasi-municipal corporation established and authorized by the state for the local administration and organization of schools.

The concept of the *intermediate unit* stems from the fact that the unit is a combination of local school districts functioning intermediately between the state department of education and the school districts providing services for both. Special districts are areas organized for specific purposes and services irrespective of other school district organizations in the area. Usually intermediate school district administration cuts across and/or bridges several local school districts.

By 1870 most states had established state boards or state organizations for the purpose of providing education. *State organization*, usually designated the state department of education, is the administrative unit usually charged with providing ongoing leadership, coordination, certification of professional staff, consultation, and monitoring and evaluation services. In addition, these agencies often serve as a linking or coordinating agent for other state and national educational agencies (Jensen and Clark, 1964).

STRUCTURE OF PUBLIC EDUCATION

Organizational structure is important because it defines the patterns of cooperation and communication between various levels of the structure and among the professional staff working in each level (Podemski et al., 1984).

Generally there are two aspects to the structure: horizontal and vertical. The vertical aspects of the structure usually represent authority levels within the school district. They can be represented schematically as is seen in Figure 5-1. (Saxe, 1975).

The more levels of vertical organization the more complex the structure and the more complicated the communication link. Podemski et al. state that:

> The vertical design for special education will specify (a) the chain of command, describing the authority relationships between subordinates and superordinates, (b) the span of control which specifies the number of individuals or departments reporting to one person, (c) the degree of centralization, the degree to which decisions and work flow are concentrated at the top of the chain of command, and (d) formalization representing the degree to which responsibilities for each position are specified in writing. Horizontal structure refers to the division of labor by which the school district combines related tasks, responsibilities, or even positions into organizational groups or divisions. The horizontal structure refers to (a) the number and responsibility of departments within the school district, and (b) the identification and assignment of tasks.

Schematic representations also depict line/staff designations. Line organization involves a direct flow of authority up and down. A line officer has direct authority over subordinates. Staff officers do not stand in a direct line of descending or ascending authority although they may at times be given *functional* authority over all aspects of the delivery of services. Generally, staff authority is assigned accord-

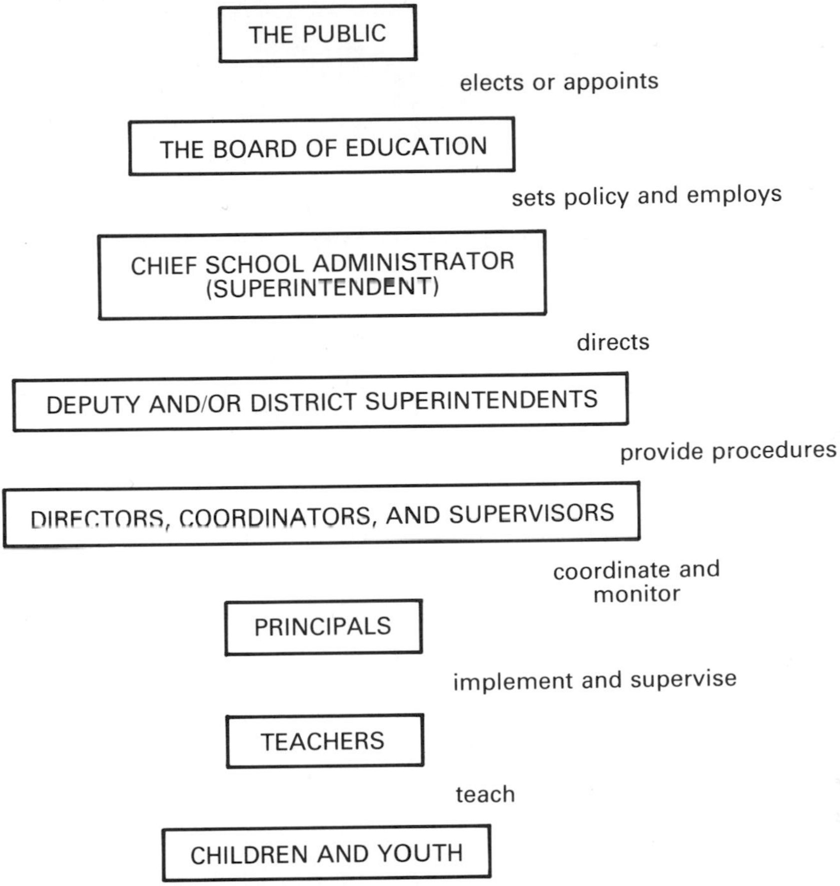

THE PUBLIC

elects or appoints

THE BOARD OF EDUCATION

sets policy and employs

CHIEF SCHOOL ADMINISTRATOR
(SUPERINTENDENT)

directs

DEPUTY AND/OR DISTRICT SUPERINTENDENTS

provide procedures

DIRECTORS, COORDINATORS, AND SUPERVISORS

coordinate and
monitor

PRINCIPALS

implement and supervise

TEACHERS

teach

CHILDREN AND YOUTH

FIGURE 5-1 Organizational Structure within the School District. *Reprinted by permission of the publisher — from Richard W. Saxe, School-Community Interaction, p. 18, figure 2.1. Copyright © 1975 by McCutchan Publishing Corporation, Berkeley, CA.*

ing to the functions they perform: service, coordinating, and advising (Negley and Evans, 1970). Figure 5-2 shows the vertical and horizontal relationships as well as line/staff relationships in a large suburban local school district.

ADMINISTRATIVE RESPONSIBILITIES FOR THE LEVELS OF AUTHORITY

The Public

American education organization has long reflected the principle of strong local control and autonomy at the district level. Therefore, the citizens of each local district are the primary source of authority for their district. Each adminis-

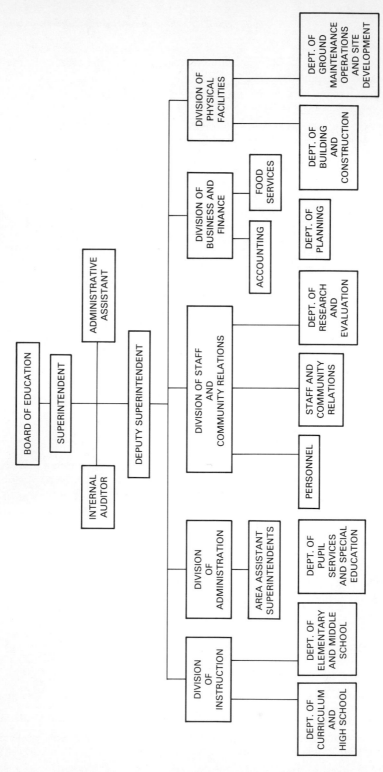

FIGURE 5-2 Relationships within a Large Suburban Local School District.

trator within the school district must then seek to involve the citizens in the educational decision-making process.

Administrators of speech-language pathology and audiology programs must actively engage in activities which inform the public of the scope and location of available services. Contacts with the public can be maintained by presentations to service organizations and P.T.A. groups and by providing for media coverage of special events (for example, national and state dates for "Speech-Language-Hearing Week").

The Board of Education

Through powers delegated to them by the state, boards of education are elected or appointed as representatives of the citizens in the management of the local school district. However, the board of education does not exercise administrative perogatives. In the main, education boards' functions include policy making; general personnel management; appointment of the superintendent; determination of programs and services; fiscal management; management of facilities at local and central levels; representing voters of the district; and representing the state in education responsibilities at the local school district level (Jensen and Clark, 1969).

Administrators of speech-language-hearing services seek opportunities to assist the board in understanding the philosophy and delivery of services to students with communication handicaps. It is not unusual for citizens to bring concerns to board members. The understanding by the board member of these services can be very helpful in providing appropriate responses to public concerns.

The Chief School Administrator (Superintendent)

The superintendent of schools is generally responsible for seeing that all laws relating to the schools, the enacted and published bylaws and policies of the state board of education, and the rules, regulations and policies of the local board of education are carried out. The superintendent is at all times subject to the control and decisions of the board of education, and usually serves as the executive officer or secretary-treasurer to the board.

Administrators of speech-language-hearing programs should endeavor to keep the superintendent of schools informed about any changes or modifications which need to be considered for more efficient and effective operation. Often the superintendent can present new ideas in such a manner as to facilitate their approval for implementation by the board of education and by the staff.

Assistant Superintendent

The assistant superintendents hold positions created by the board of education to assist the superintendent of schools in the operation of the school system. The duties of the assistant superintendents include:

- executive direction, control and evaluation of the system-wide program of education

- acting as principal advisor to the superintendent in the administration of schools and the implementation of the education program
- coordination of the activities of directors and supervisors
- preparation and/or coordination of the preparation of policies and procedures related to the education program
- coordination of the staff relationship with local school administrators
- coordination of the services of their assigned departments as they function in the individual schools.

Administrators of speech-language and audiology services utilize assistant superintendents to provide endorsement for and facilitation of procedures for conducting speech pathology and audiology programs with school principals.

Directors, Coordinators, Supervisors

Directors, coordinators and supervisors are responsible to the superintendent of schools for the overall improvement, maintenance and coordination of the educational program. In general their duties are assigned by the superintendent and/or the staff for the purpose of achieving the following objectives:

- translating the school system's educational goals into the educational program
- reporting the extent of the achievement of these goals
- recommending to the superintendent of schools appropriate policies, regulations and procedures to eliminate any discovered weakness in the achievement of goals for their assigned areas of responsibility.

Administrators of speech-language-hearing programs usually occupy this middle-management level.

Principals

Principals are appointed by the board of education upon recommendation of the superintendent. The duties of principals are to:

- serve as the administrative head of the local school with the responsibility for all activities that occur there
- focus primary attention on the supervision and improvement of instruction
- report directly to the appropriate assistant superintendent or to the superintendent
- utilize all central staff and local school personnel to assist in the operation of the school
- evaluate the effectiveness of personnel assigned to the facility
- inform the superintendent or staff of community issues or concerns.

Administrators of speech-language-hearing programs work cooperatively with principals to implement the therapy services in each school. Establishing positive interactions and interweaving the responsibilities of both administrators are vital to the delivery of quality services. Sensitivity to and understanding of the philosophies of education and clinical approaches will enhance these relationships.

Understanding of an organizational structure and line/staff relationships is vital if an administrator of speech-language-hearing services is to provide efficient and effective leadership. Since the structures have already been established and have been operating over significant periods of time, the administrator of the speech-language-hearing services program must be able to apply this knowledge and understanding to identify:

- the most efficient and effective path to accomplish desired changes in the provision of services
- the most effective means of coalescing resources to support quality services
- the most effective path to circumvent the dysfunctional aspects of the organization or education delivery system

ORGANIZATIONAL STRUCTURE AND THE SPEECH-LANGUAGE-HEARING SERVICES PROGRAM

In the vertical aspects of organization the person administering the speech-language-hearing services program is not in a line relationship but generally occupies a staff position. The administrator is usually directly responsible to a district assistant superintendent, director of a department, or coordinator of a program.

In the horizontal aspects of organization the speech-language-hearing services are designated as a service within an office or department which relates directly to instruction. Most frequently these services can be found within the department of special education or the department of pupil services. The purpose of the department of special education is to organize and administer instruction and related services so that each educationally handicapped child in the district is provided a free appropriate public education program in the least restrictive environment. The purpose of the department of pupil services is to provide support services to all students in the district to overcome any internal or external (home/community) problems they may experience. Pupil personnel services usually include psychological services, guidance services, nursing services, and social services.

The administration, departmental interaction, and day-to-day operation of these services is impacted upon by the locus of control of the organization's decision-making process. Some school organizations subscribe to a centralized model of administration and decision making. In this case the administrator of speech-language-hearing services exerts substantial influence in coordinating and monitoring services as they are delivered in all schools in the district.

In other locations the district operates under a decentralized model whereby the local school administrator is granted a significant amount of authority in deciding how programs and services are to be conducted in his or her facility. When this occurs the administrator for speech-language-hearing services often serves in a consultative, coordinating, facilitative role to the local school administrator.

Organizational structures are sometimes influenced by size and geographic locations. Administrative operations, and decision-making prerogatives of administrators of speech-language-hearing programs are quite different when these services are provided in large school districts, medium-sized districts, and rural districts. In each setting the administrator for speech-language-hearing services must take into account the unique characteristics of that setting and the nature of its organizational structure. There are advantages and disadvantages associated with each of the three. Some of these characteristics have been identified as they apply to the provision of special education services to handicapped pupils (Podemski et al., 1984). They also are relevant to provision of speech-language-hearing services. These characteristics, for the purpose of this chapter, have been modified to address speech-language-hearing services. They are presented in Table 5-1.

TABLE 5-1   Advantages and Disadvantages Associated with Provision of Speech-Hearing-Language Services

	ADVANTAGES	DISADVANTAGES
Local School System (Urban Districts, County School Systems)	Sufficient number of speech-language-hearing handicapped students to offer organized comprehensive services	Coordination activities between central office and local schools is more difficult due to numbers and distance
	Designated administrative and support staff to facilitate operations and provide assistance to local SLP's and audiologists	Horizontal integration among departmental units is more complex and communication breakdowns are enhanced
	Well established comprehensive policies, procedures, goals, objectives	Diverse "publics" produce wide spectrums of expectations as to the need and nature of speech-language-hearing services
	Specialized units to deal with unique populations and with different age groups	Effective integration of centralized and decentralized administrative functions is difficult to achieve
	Formalized authority structure which specifies line of responsibility and communication	Limited fiscal resources distributed across many departments
	Other public and private agencies which can provide or augment lacking diagnostic and treatment services	
Medium Sized Districts (2,500–10,000 Students) 33% of School-Age Children in U.S.	Community stability provides opportunity for better understanding and support for broad spectrum of services including speech-language-hearing	Smaller school populations may require unique staffing patterns to provide appropriate speech-hearing-language services
	Organizational structure and administrative activities are less complex and the distance between those	Staff/pupil ratios may be higher resulting in higher per pupil cost
		Multiple school assignments may result in reduction of level and

	who organize and those who deliver speech-language-hearing services is smaller Coordination of implementing and monitoring speech-language-hearing services delivery enhances quality of service	frequency of speech-hearing-language services Higher dependence on community diagnostic and treatment resources Needed supplementary community resources may be unavailable or their location may be significantly removed from source of need School systems may need to contract with outside agencies or other school districts to provide services Problems of vertical and horizontal integration are increased
Rural Districts 54% of School Districts in U.S. 8% of Country's School Population	Close to community administrators well-known to residents Close personal speech-language pathologist relationships	Small incidence of speech-language-hearing handicap results in multiple school assignments which impact on frequency of contact Community may not view speech-language-hearing services as important, causing low levels of parental involvement Geographic and climatic factors may affect consistency of service Low tax base, low financial levels of support may exist Difficulty in recruiting certified staff Educational organization limitations
Intermediate or Cooperative School Districts 35 States Have Some Form	Pooled resources facilitate offering speech-language-hearing services which a single school district may not afford More specialized staff: Speech-language pathologists and audiologists can be employed Services can be provided to low incidence handicapped populations Improved organization and administration Administration and supervision can be shared	Community identity of individualized service delivery is valued Cooperative interactions among school administrators and teachers across districts is sometimes difficult to manage Services across distances cause problems in travel and communication Lines of authority are blurred and communication channels are unclear Funding sources and equalization among cooperating districts can be a source of friction Political considerations become a factor in service delivery

THE SPEECH-LANGUAGE-HEARING PROGRAM
IN A PUBLIC SCHOOL SETTING

The speech-language-hearing program is an integral part of the general education program of a public school system. Much of a student's success in school and in the community depends on how well the student can give expression to ideas and emotions. Modern society places a high value upon skill in communication and demands for this skill are constantly increasing.

The concept underlying the speech-language-hearing programs in public schools is the selection and application of scientific techniques to meet the needs of a specific child who is manifesting receptive and/or expressive deviations in communication. The alleviation of the symptoms depends upon the appropriateness of the techniques in relation to the child as well as to the disorder, and upon the quality of the therapeutic relationship (Baltimore County Public Schools Workshop Staff, 1965).

The administration of speech-language must seek support for the inclusion of both speech pathology and audiology service and provide an operational system that will assure their availability. The organization, administration and delivery of speech pathology and audiology services in public schools must be based on a commitment (a) to provide comprehensive services of the highest quality to all students, 0 years to 21 years, with communication disabilities; (b) to make available to these students a full range of consultative, assessment, and clinical services; (c) to provide individualized therapeutic programs for students who require intervention because of breakdowns in the communication process; (d) to use a repertoire of clinical techniques and approaches in keeping with current scientific knowledge in the fields of speech, language, and hearing science; (e) to disseminate to parents, school personnel and citizens in the community information regarding the need for early identification and the availability of service for children and youth with speech, hearing and/or language disorders; and to (f) maintain a clinical program of high quality which stimulates and provides for professional growth and development of those who provide therapeutic services (Baltimore County Public Schools Workshop Staff, 1982). In addition, it must endorse the preservation of the highest standards of integrity and ethical principles, which are vital to the successful discharge of professional responsibilities of all speech-language-hearing pathologists and audiologists (American Speech-Language-Hearing Association Code of Ethics, 1979).

Further, the administrative design must provide policies and procedures which assure monitoring of the quality of the speech-language-hearing services and compliance with federal and state mandates.

General Administrative Structure

Speech-language-hearing services are generally depicted as being a service provided through the division of instruction or through the division of pupil services. When associated with the division of instruction the schematic representation of vertical horizontal relationships may be shown as in Figure 5-3. The entire organi-

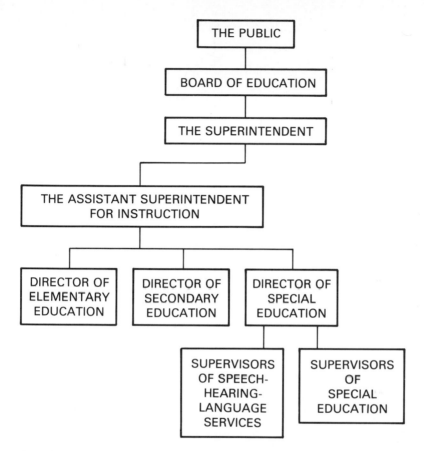

FIGURE 5-3 Speech-Language-Hearing Services as Related to the Division
of Instruction.

zation tree is not provided, just the aspect relating directly to the division of instruction.

Under this arrangement the alignment with instruction reinforces the district's concept that the speech-language-hearing services are an integral part of the instructional process and educational offering.

When associated with the department of pupil services the administrative design supports the school system perception that speech-language-hearing services are one of several support services which are related to instruction but not necessarily an integral part of them. This arrangement is seen in Figure 5–4.

Sometimes a model for administration shows that both instructional and support services are combined under one administrative head. Figure 5–5 shows a schematic representation of this model.

This model highlights the equality of instructional services for nonhandicapped and handicapped students and supports the concept that special education, pupil

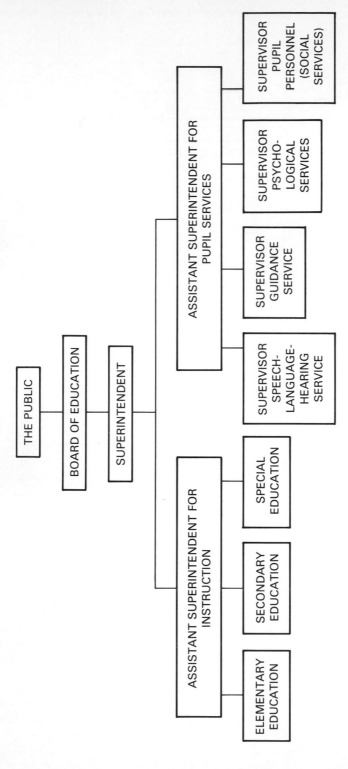

FIGURE 5-4 Speech-Language-Hearing Services as Related to Pupil Services.

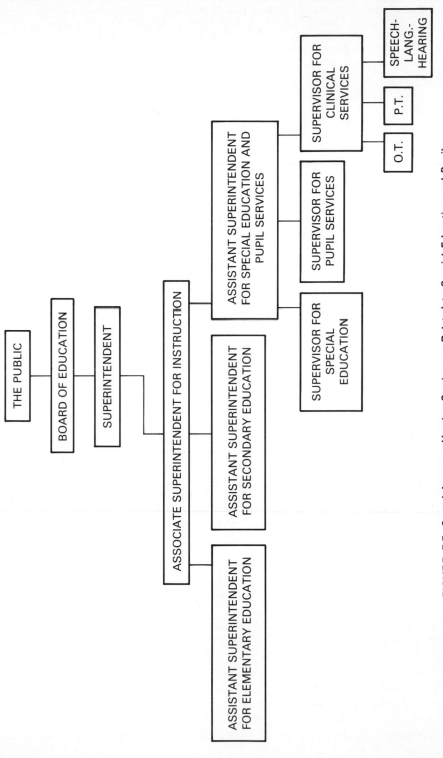

FIGURE 5-5 Speech-Language-Hearing Services as Related to Special Education and Pupil Services.

services, and clinical services are integrated within one department but all three are amalgamated under one administrator who has direct access to the associate superintendent for instruction.

Each school system has its own schematic representation. Each design presents aspects which facilitate and to a limited degree impede program operation. It must be remembered, however, that school systems are organized to carry out an instructional program for students. All other programs are viewed as adjunctive. The administrator of the speech-language-hearing program must be realistic and flexible, and must be aware and sensitive to the idiosyncracies in organization from one program or system to another (Van Hattum, 1969).

THE ALL HANDICAPPED CHILDRENS ACT (P.L. 94-142)
AND THE ADMINISTRATION
OF SPEECH-LANGUAGE-HEARING PROGRAMS

The All Handicapped Childrens Act (P.L. 94-142) has had a pervasive effect on how states and local education agencies organize and administer services to handicapped children, including those with communication disorders. Since its passage in 1975 the following changes have occurred at the state level.

- All states have passed enabling legislation which coincides with P.L. 94-142 and its regulations.
- Policies and procedures at both the state and local levels have been revised and published to assure compliance with the regulations.
- The role of administrators at the state level has changed from an advisory consultative responsibility to that of monitoring, to ensure that the provisions of state and federal regulations are met.
- The state education agencies channel funds for the implementation of P.L. 94-142 to the local education agencies.
- The state departments of education are charged with preparing and submitting annual program plans.
- The state education agencies channel funds for the implementation of P.L. 94-142 to the local education agencies.
- The state departments of education are charged with preparing and submitting annual program plans in order to receive federal funds for the education of handicapped students.
- The state departments of education are monitored and evaluated by representatives of the federal office charged with implementing the law to assure that the state is in compliance with federal regulations for the handicapped.

The local school districts are also impacted upon by the law. The administrator of speech-language-hearing programs must see that these services are in compliance with (1) the general requirements of the law, and (2) those requirements that relate specifically to the speech-language-hearing handicapped.

General Requirements

The regulations of P.L. 94-142 refer to the processes of identification, assessment, educational decision, educational placement, and due process. In order to be in compliance, the administrator of speech-language-hearing services must:

- develop and implement "child find" procedures to assure that every communication-handicapped child or youth who lives in the district is identified
- provide and arrange for each child or youth suspected of having a communication handicap to be assessed using nondiscriminatory procedures and instruments
- arrange for a process that supports an interdisciplinary team consideration of the assessment information so that a free appropriate public education and/or related services program can be provided
- assure that a continuum of services, from least to most intense, be made available and that they be provided in the least restrictive educational setting
- require that an individualized education program (I.E.P.) addressing the assessed needs of each communicatively handicapped child be developed and written with the participation of the child's or youth's parents
- provide for and monitor the implementation of the "due process" rights of the child or youth and the parents. These rights include the right to examine records; to obtain an independent evaluation; to receive prior notice before an assessment or a change in I.E.P. or program; and to disagree with and appeal (at local, state and district court level) a decision made by the school district
- provide access to related services including transportation and such developmental and corrective services as may be required to assist the child to benefit from the educational program.

Requirements Related
to Speech-Language-Hearing Impaired

P.L. 94-142 addresses the speech-language-hearing impaired by (1) providing definitions to assure consistency as to the individuals determined to be handicapped under the provisions of the law (section 300a.5); (2) describing who are considered "qualified examiners" to determine the presence of a handicapping condition (section 300a.531); (3) providing for accessibility to direct related services (sections 300a.13 and 300a.14); (4) supporting proper functioning of hearing aids (300a.303); (5) describing conditions for preplacement evaluation (300a.531(P)); and (6) specifying conditions pertaining to placement decisions (300a.533, "comment").

Administrators of speech-language-hearing programs must familiarize themselves with the requirements of these sections and diligently monitor the day-to-day operations to assure that they are understood by local school administrators and professional staff and that they are being put into effect. They must prepare their staff and local school personnel for compliance reviews which are conducted by state departments of education and/or the U.S. Office of Education: Special Education.

ADMINISTRATIVE RESPONSIBILITIES INVOLVED IN THE PUBLIC SCHOOL SETTING

State Department of Education

Organization for the purposes of assuring the provision of speech, language, and audiology services may reflect a categorical or noncategorical arrangement. A noncategorical organization reflects a regional design which emphasizes the assignment of one administrator per region within the state who is responsible for the delivery of services for handicapped students across all categories of handicapping conditions. Statewide monitoring of speech-language-hearing programs is just one of the programs for which the administrator is responsible. Often this administrator has little training or experience in providing clinical services.

Sometimes this administrative design assigns the administrator both administrative and program responsibilities. If this is the case, then each administrator is charged with cross-categorical responsibilities and a program (for example, speech-language pathology/audiology, learning disabilities, or vision) consultation responsibility. When this design is used, the regional administrator who holds program responsibility for speech-language-hearing services is called upon to provide consultation to other regional administrators or to local school district personnel.

If the state department of education is organized to reflect categorical responsibilities, the administrator for speech-language-hearing services usually is trained and certified in speech-language pathology and/or audiology and provides monitoring and consultation of these specific services to all regions within the state.

In general, state department consultants for speech-language-hearing services do the following:

- provide consultation to all counties and school systems requesting assistance
- plan and assist in conducting district, county, regional, or statewide conferences and inservice training
- develop and submit for approval requirements for the certification of speech-language pathologists and audiologists
- promote the establishment of sound professional criteria for conducting speech-language pathology and audiology services in the school districts across the state
- monitor and evaluate the quality of services to assure legal compliance, identify areas of weakness, and provide suggestions for improvement utilizing available state resources
- interpret federal and state regulations and inform local school districts of any changes in regulations
- work closely with colleges and universities to improve training of speech-language pathologists and audiologists
- coordinate information and speech-language pathology and audiology needs in the state and communicate this information to administrators of divisions within the state department of education (Van Hattum, 1969).

Intermediate School District

The duties and responsibilities of an administrator at the intermediate school district level bear direct correspondence to the established purposes the district was designed to accomplish. If the intermediate school district is established to provide an umbrella under which the services to the handicapped are coordinated, then the administrative role will be related to:

- planning and conducting professional conferences and inservice training opportunities for speech-language pathologists in participating school districts
- serving as intermediary in interpreting state department standards and regulations
- working with the various participating district administrators to analyze and improve the quality of speech pathology and audiology services across districts
- providing consultative service to administrators in participating districts
- coordinating research projects and/or program evaluation efforts
- coordinating available school and community resources to provide appropriate service in districts where service offerings are less than comprehensive.

If the intermediate school district assumes responsibility for the actual provision of speech pathology and/or audiology services for participating school districts, then the responsibilities of the administrator will be involved with the direction, supervision and communication related to speech pathology and/or audiology services (Freeman, 1969). The administrative duties may include:

- organizing and conducting a central diagnostic and treatment center for students with severe speech, language, and hearing disabilities, who cannot be appropriately served in any one school district
- providing information to the sending school district and descriptions of the impact of the speech-, language-, and hearing-impaired student upon educational management
- providing treatment/education management plans to be implemented at the school district level by district personnel
- providing supplemental and consultative assistance to local school districts.

School District

The management responsibilities associated with the operation of speech-language pathology and audiology services are twofold: administrative and supervisory. Some administrative and supervisory tasks are clearly assigned to the individual appointed as administrator of speech pathology and audiology services; other administrative and supervisory duties are shared between the administrator and the school principal.

ADMINISTRATIVE AND SUPERVISORY TASKS
ASSOCIATED WITH PUBLIC SCHOOL PROGRAMS
OF SPEECH PATHOLOGY AND AUDIOLOGY

First and foremost, the administrator for speech-language pathology and audiology must identify and specify the scope of these services and must clearly articulate procedures for acquiring and conducting these services at both the central staff and local administrative levels. The development and distribution of a resource manual for use as a reference by central staff, local school principals, and speech-language pathologists and audiologists generally facilitates the understanding and implementation of these services. The resource manual can cover such areas as:

- philosophy of the speech-language and audiology program
- purpose and use of the resource guide
- administration of the speech pathology/audiology program

    administrative responsibilities of the coordinator/supervisor
    administrative responsibilities of the principal
    operational procedures for speech-language pathology services
    operational procedures for audiological services
    role and responsibilities of speech-language pathologist
    role and responsibilities of audiologist
    role and responsibilities of school nurse
    role and responsibilities of the consulting physician
    role and responsibilities of the classroom teacher
    role and responsibilities of the teacher of the hearing impaired
    role and responsibilities of support personnel (aides)

- operational procedures

    organization at school level
    case selection process (identification, assessment, interdisciplinary team decision)
    I.E.P. production
    scheduling procedures
    reporting
    clinical management
    conferences
    physical plant
    equipment and materials

- related and support services
- community resources

Thirdly, the administrator of speech-language pathology and audiology services must clearly articulate the goals and objectives of the services. These goals and objectives should address: (a) the unique aspect of clinical intervention as it relates to individuals and (b) the instructional resource aspect of consultation. Training and experience in such areas as language acquisition and competent performance can be an important resource that should be accessed by those charged with curriculum development.

A fourth administrative task is essential for the provision of speech-language pathology and audiology service. This task involves budget preparation and management. A budget is a plan for the allocation of fiscal resources to various programs within the organization over a specified period of time. The yearly budget period may be either calendar or fiscal. The calendar year begins January 1 and ends on December 31; and the fiscal year for schools refers to the school year, July 1–June 30. Since federal fiscal support is a factor in calculating resources, those responsible for fiscal development must also be cognizant of the federal fiscal year, October 1–September 30.

The school district determines the basic budgeting method to be used. Some methods used by school districts include program planning and budget systems (PPBS), zero-based budgeting, and the school planning, evaluation and communication system (SPECS). All of these systems are based on the concept that the budget is broken down into specific programs and parts of programs so that funds expended can be traced to program results (Podemski et al., 1984).

The administrator for speech-language-hearing services has responsibility for (1) determining program needs based on information provided by principals, instructional specialists, and school-based speech-language pathologists and audiologists; (2) organizing the requests according to the budget system selected by the school system; (3) providing support data and justification statements for the requested resources; and (4) submitting the request to the appropriate line officers for their review and revision. Further, the administrator should attend and be prepared to explain and justify the requests before the community and the board of education during budget hearings.

A fifth important administrative task is to assure that services of the highest quality are provided to speech-language-hearing-impaired students. One way that this can be done is for the administrator to ensure the employment of certified competent speech-language pathologists and audiologists. Depending on the size of the school system, organizational complexities, and role/responsibility decisions, the administrator for speech-language pathology may or may not be directly involved in the recruitment, interview, and employment process. However, the administrator, by establishing good communication with those responsible for employment, can influence and persuade them to identify and select those speech-language pathologists and audiologists with the best credentials. The administrator should:

- direct recruiter attention to facilities recognized by the profession as providing training of the highest quality
- volunteer to accompany recruiters to training institutions
  identify time periods when applications are received
- review the applications to see that academic credentials meet requirements

for Certificate of Clinical Competence in Speech Pathology or Audiology and inform the personnel representatives of prioritized choices

- volunteer to participate in applicant interviews and ask predesigned questions to confirm clinical competence
- arrange for candidates to visit schools in the assignment schedule so that principal's input can be secured.

Another activity which assists in supporting the provision of quality service is the administrator's active participation in the certification process. Educational systems have long been involved in establishing standards for professional competency. While careful consideration is given to establishing standards that address effective instruction, less attention has been paid to establishing standards addressing competencies of other professionals providing services different from instruction. Since states set standards, the certification standards for speech-language pathologists may emanate from standards established by state departments of education, standards established by state licensure boards, or both. Administrators then must be familiar with the basis for the established standards, and with how closely they match the professional standards. Where certification standards are lower than professional standards, the administrator must convince the state Department of Education and the school system administrators that the professional standards are the only acceptable ones. Administrators must insist that the personnel representatives seek only candidates who hold a Certificate of Clinical Competence in Speech or Audiology, or qualify for a Clinical Fellowship Year experience.

School systems have for too long accepted a standard based on teaching competency standards. If a high value is placed by the school system on quality teachers, the administrator must work to achieve the same commitment for speech pathologists and audiologists.

Administrators can assure quality service through selecting and implementing program study and evaluation procedures. Several mechanisms for quality assurance have been described in the literature. These include:

1. PDME: Planning, Development, Management, Evaluation
   This is a systems management approach which involves the collecting, analyzing, disseminating and revising of essential information to aid in policy formation and administrative decision making (Jones and Healey, 1973). A manual is available to provide assistance in implementation.
2. CSRS: Child Services Review System
   This quality-assurance strategy is designed to measure documents and improve the quality of speech-language-hearing and special education procedures. Utilizing a retrospective peer review process, speech-language pathologists and audiologists conduct a CSRS audit. Implementation of this system depends upon an intensive series of workshops that rely on small group dynamics and experiential learning. Participants perform steps of the audit sequence and simulate audits for two different problems using pupil records (Barnes and Pines, 1982).
3. PCAS: Patient-Care Audit System
   This method of process assessment focuses on client services and uses peer

analysis of client records. The retrospective audit allows for the review of past service to provide the basis for future practice. The Patient-Care Audit System incorporates a series of sequential activities that involve (a) selection of an aspect of patient care for review, (b) establishment of standards of quality within the area, (c) retrospective review of selected client charts according to the standards, and (d) identification of patterns of care (Adair and Griffin, 1979).

4. Professional Services Board Accreditation

This process features quality-of-service analysis based on confirmation through site visit that the school system's actual policies and procedures adhere to the standards for the provision of service established by the American Speech-Language-Hearing Association. A certificate of accreditation is awarded to inform the public that the services provided are of the highest quality. This program evaluation service is accessible by submitting an application to the Professional Services Board of the American Speech-Language-Hearing Association (ASHA, Public Services Board Standards, 1983).

SUPERVISORY ASPECTS OF ADMINISTRATION

The supervisory aspect of administration is the most important responsibility the administrator fulfills. One component of this responsibility refers to program management; the other component refers to clinical management.

Program management activities involve the supervision of the general operating process and procedures. This duty is usually shared by local building administrators and the administrator for speech-language-hearing services. Working together, the administrators will monitor such activities as (1) staff assignment time, (Full Time Equivalent assignment), (2) ordering and distribution of equipment and material, (3) program/services planning and scheduling, (4) compliance with state and federal regulations, (5) attendance, (6) faculty/pathologist/audiologist interaction, and (7) parent/pathologist/audiologist interactions.

Supervision of clinical operations occupies most of the assigned work time for the administrator of speech-language-hearing services. There are three areas that are addressed in the process: (1) implementation of the goals and objectives of the speech pathology and audiology services program in each school; (2) observation and evaluation of personnel; and (3) case consultation.

School administrators and the administrator for speech-language pathology and audiology services usually share responsibilities for the first two areas. The local school administrator can provide insight into the efficiency of the day-to-day operation; information about the relevance of the services provided to the overall goals and objectives of the program; and perceptions of students', parents', and teachers' reactions to the service.

Many school systems have now adopted a team approach to observation and evaluation. Administrators of speech pathology and audiology programs must be informed about and sensitive to the fact that the process may be based on "master agreements" between teachers' associations or unions and boards of education.

Again, when evaluation responsibilities are shared, participants usually agree as to which aspect of professional performance each is qualified to address. The principal's evaluation usually contributes information related to an educational perspective. Some areas of performance may include:

1. Professional Competencies
   knowledge of the student, knowledge of subject matter
   planning and program implementation
   evidence of professional growth activities
   motivation of students
   communication skills
2. Human Relations Competencies
   rapport with students
   intergroup relationships (teacher/administrator, supervisory)
   relationship with parents
3. Management Competencies
   pupil control
   reporting practices
   appearance/room organization
   dependability

Supervision from the standpoint of the administrator of speech pathology and audiology services refers to the tasks of clinical teaching related to the interaction between clinician and client. Thirteen tasks basic to effective clinical teaching, comprising the distinct area of practice which constitute clinical supervision in communication, have been identified through the cumulative effort of several members of the American Speech-Language-Hearing Association and the Committee on Supervision in Speech-Language Pathology and Audiology (ASHA: Clinical Supervision, 1984).

"The tasks of supervision include:

1. establishing and maintaining an effective working relationship with the supervisee
2. assisting the supervisee in developing goals and objectives
3. assisting the supervisee in developing and refining assessment skills
4. assisting the supervisee in developing and refining clinical management skills
5. demonstrating or participating with the supervisee in the clinical process
6. assisting the supervisee in observing and analyzing assessment and treatment sessions
7. assisting the supervisee in the development and maintenance of clinical and supervisory records
8. interacting with the supervisee in planning, executing, and analyzing supervisory conferences
9. assisting the supervisee in evaluation of clinical performances
10. assisting the supervisee in developing skills of verbal reporting, writing, and editing

11. sharing information regarding ethical, legal, regulatory, and reimbursement aspects of professional practice
12. modeling professional conduct
13. demonstrating research skills in the clinical or supervisory processes."

While engaging in these tasks and observing the supervisee's response to them, evaluation reports as to the level of competent performance for each speech-language pathologist and audiologist can be generated by the administrator for speech pathology and audiology services.

SUGGESTIONS TO FUTURE SPEECH-LANGUAGE-HEARING ADMINISTRATORS IN A PUBLIC SCHOOL SETTING

For those contemplating a career change from speech-language pathologist or audiologist to administration of these programs, several factors should be examined. First, those interested in administration must determine the responsibilities associated with the position and match them to their personal goals and objectives. There are positive and negative aspects associated with administration. While salary and prestige may be viewed as pluses, encroachment of responsibilities on personal free time and family responsibilities may be viewed as minuses. It is therefore suggested that the individual determine (1) the degree of satisfaction to be derived from examining current organization and operation, and planning for modification to be phased in over a period of time; (2) the degree of satisfaction to be derived from guiding and challenging adults to achieve; (3) the degree of satisfaction to be derived from efforts directed toward program development rather than from endeavors related to clinical management; (4) the degree of patience that must be expended in assisting the various "publics" with which the administrator must interact; and (5) the breadth of strategies that must be developed to cope with stress emanating from unrealized goals, shortened time lines, and staffing problems.

If the conclusion drawn from self-examination is that administration presents a positive challenge, a second factor must then be addressed. The potential candidate for administration must become a master clinician. Professional training in speech-language pathology and/or audiology which complies with standards required for the Certificate of Clinical Competence in speech pathology and/or audiology is essential. In addition, the candidate must be employed in a public school in order to gain client-clinician experience, knowledge about the organization and operation of the program on a day-to-day basis, information based on experience of the problems and the rewards associated with provision of speech, language, and hearing services in school environments, and information about administration of programs based on direct observation.

A third factor which impacts upon an individual's goal to become an administrator refers to professional preparation for administration. The candidate must meet professional competency requirements in administration.

The profession of speech-language pathology and audiology has developed some recommended guidelines for supervision (ASHA Minimum Qualifications, 1982). Though they have not been adopted by certifying bodies (that is, state departments of education), they are offered here for informational purposes.

1. The master's degree or equivalent in the subject area (speech-language pathology or audiology) for which supervision will be provided
2. The Certificate of Clinical Competence in the subject area (speech-language pathology or audiology) for which supervision will be provided
3. At least two years of full-time professional experience beyond the Clinical Fellowship Year in the subject area (speech-language pathology or audiology) to be supervised
4. Coursework in supervision consisting of at least six semester credit hours or nine continuing education units, or some combination thereof, applicable to the supervisory process, of which at least one-half must be specific to the supervisory process in communication disorders
5. Practicum in supervision. At least fifty clock hours of practicum experience in supervising the provision of direct services to clients must be obtained following completion of the Clinical Fellowship Year.

Professionals seeking appointment to administrative or supervisory positions should realize that they must meet certification requirements for speech pathology and/or audiology, and certification requirements for administration and supervision, which have been established by state departments of education.

Many state departments of education describe administration certification requirements as part of a general administration credential or as a special education administration credential. The following components are reviewed before a certificate is issued:

- eligibility for a professional certificate appropriate to the assignment (for example, speech pathology)
- a master's degree from an accredited institution
- a specified number of semester hours of graduate credit beyond the master's degree

If the credential is issued as part of special education, and because administrative assignments are often designed to include delivery of special education instructional service, the future administrator should enroll in special education courses which develop the following:

- competence in the development, selection, administration, and interpretation of formal and informal assessment techniques to assess a child's *educational* development focusing on normal growth and development and the implications of deviations from these patterns
- competence in the development, implementation and evaluation of a variety of sequentially ordered instructional approaches for exceptional children which accommodate their academic, social, cognitive, and physical needs

- competence in describing the characteristics of each exceptionality and their effects on how children learn
- competence in planning and evaluating individualized educational programs for handicapped children
- an understanding of national, state, and local laws, policies and procedures affecting the handicapped and developing a system for organizing and maintaining student records (Content standards 3.5.12, Exceptional Handicapped Children, 1983).

A fourth factor which impacts on the goal of becoming an administrator of a speech, language, hearing services program is the administration selection process established by the school district. Many of the larger school districts have developed and offer leadership training. Currently those individuals interested in being appointed as administrators must complete this training and participate in the process of selection based on structured interview. Information pertaining to this training and selection is usually available through personnel departments.

A fifth factor which often has direct bearing upon appointment to an administration position concerns the applicant's direct and in-depth knowledge of the current organization and procedures for delivering a systemwide program of speech pathology and/or audiology services. In many school systems, negotiated agreements require that administration vacancies be advertised throughout the district in which the vacancy exists and in other surrounding districts. Those applying for such positions should take time to investigate the organization, the administrative design, the responsibilities of the position, and the appropriateness of their own training and philosophy regarding the provision of service. Applicants should anticipate questions relating to the administrative responsibilities and be prepared to describe what they would do to maintain or improve services, if appointed.

The sixth factor is persistence. Often school districts have a number of candidates for administrative positions, all of whom present comparable credentials. Therefore, potential administrators should be prepared to submit their credentials and applications each time a vacancy for which they are qualified occurs. Each time a candidate for an administrative position participates in the selection process, he or she learns more from the experience, in terms of organization and presentation of ideas. As the applicant becomes more familiar with the process, he or she gains confidence. In addition, the candidate should schedule a follow-up meeting with one of the members of the interview committee to determine the strengths and/or weaknesses of the interview.

SUMMARY

Educational environments with positive attitudinal supports from students, parents, and teachers provide a viable setting for the provision of quality speech-pathology and audiology services. Unlike other environments, public schools have local, state, and federal mandates to provide the philosophical and financial support to offer free appropriate services.

Several factors assist those charged with the management of speech, language, and audiology programs in public schools.

- There is an established organization which provides a ready-made arrangement for management. It is essential that those charged with operational responsibilities be knowledgeable about the administrative hierarchy, and the process by which goals are established and objectives achieved.
- There are federal and state regulations which establish the character and monitor the provision of services to handicapped students. Therefore, the monitoring role of these agencies provide the vehicle and incentive for administrators of speech-language pathology and audiology services to arrange program evaluation systems that assure quality.
- There are established criteria for training and certification for administrators, and these form the foundation for consideration for employment. Those seeking administrative positions must be trained, experienced, and prepared to offer skills and experience which will assure competent performance.

REFERENCES

ADAIR, M. N., AND K. N. GRIFFIN. (1979). "Quality assurance: A professional quest for speech-language pathologists and audiologists," *Asha*, 21, 871–874.

AINSWORTH, S. H. (1959). "Identity and identification," *Asha*, 1, 11–12.

AMERICAN SPEECH-LANGUAGE-HEARING ASSOCIATION. (1978). "Current status of supervision of speech-language pathology and audiology (special report)," *Asha*, 20, 478–486.

———. (1982). "Minimal qualifications for supervisors and suggested competencies for effective clinical supervision (draft)," *Asha*, 24, 339–342.

———. (1982). "Suggested competencies for effective clinical supervision," *Asha*, 24, 1021–1023.

———. (1982). "Responses to proposed qualifications for supervisors," *Asha*, 24, 1025–1029.

———. "Ad hoc committee on extension of audiological services in schools report (1983). Audiology Services in the Schools (position statement)," *Asha*, 25, 53–59.

———. (1983). "New standards for accreditation by the professional services board," *Asha*, 26(6), 51–58.

———. (1984). Committee on rehabilitative audiology report: Definition of and competencies for aural rehabilitation (position statement)," *Asha*, 26, 37–41.

———. (1984). "Clinical supervision (draft statements)," *Asha*, 26, 45–48.

BARNES, K. J., AND P. L. PINES. (1982). "Assessing and improving services to the handicapped," *Asha*, 24, 555–559.

BLAIR, J. C., AND F. S. BERG. (1982). "Problems and needs of hard of hearing students and a model for the delivery of services to the schools," *Asha*, 24, 541–545.

BLANCHARD, M. M. AND E. H. NOBER. (1978). "The impact of state and federal legislation on public school speech-language-hearing clinicians," *Speech Language Hearing Services in Schools*, 2, 77–84.

BRUBAKER, K. L. and R. H. NELSON, (1974). *Creative survival in educational bureaucracies.* Berkeley, Cal.: McCutchan Publishing Corp.

CACCAMO, J. M. (1974). "Speech, language and audiological services—An inalienable right," *Language, Speech and Hearing Services in Schools*, 5, 173–175.

CAUSEY, L. M., K. D., JOHNSON, AND W. C. HEALEY. (1971). "A survey of state certification requirements for public school speech clinicians," *Asha*, 13, 123–129.

CRICHTON, L. J., AND A. R. ORATIO. (1984). "Speech-Language Pathologists' Clinical Fellowship Training," *Asha*, 26, 39–43.

DOUGLASS, R. L. (1983). "Clinical accountability: Schools, clinics, private practice," *Seminars in Speech and Language*, 4, 107–185.

DUBLINSKE, S. (1978). "Special reports, P.L. 94-142: Developing the individualized education program (I.E.P.)," *Asha*, 20,393-397.
FEIN, D. J. (1983). "Prevalence of speech and language impairments," *Asha*, 24, 37-38.
———. (1983). "Population data from the U.S. census bureau," *Asha*, 25, 53-57.
———. (1983). "Survey report: 1982 ASHA omnibus," *Asha*, 25, 53-57.
———. (1984). "Findings from the 1983 omnibus survey," *Asha*, 26, 45-48.
FREEMAN, G. G. (1969). "Innovative school programs: The Oakland schools plan," *Journal of Speech and Hearing Disorders*, 34, 220-225.
GROSS, F. P., AND G. R. FICHTER. (1970). "Professional negotiations and the school speech and hearing clinician," *Asha*, 12, 124-126.
HEALEY, W. C. (1973-1974). *Standards and Guidelines for Comprehensive Language Speech, and Hearing Problems in Schools*. Rockville, Md.: American Speech and Hearing Association.
IMPLEMENTATION OF PART B OF THE EDUCATION OF THE HANDICAPPED ACT. (1977). *Federal Register*, 42, 42474-42518.
IRWIN, R. B. (1959). "Speech therapy in the public schools: State legislation and certification," *Journal of Speech and Hearing Services in Schools*, 24, 127.
———. (1976). "Speech and hearing therapy in the public schools in Ohio," *Journal of Speech and Hearing Disorders*, 14, 63-68.
JENSEN, T. J., AND D. L. CLARK. (1964). *Educational administration*. New York: The Center For Applied Research In Education, Inc.
JONES, S., AND W. C. HEALEY. (1973). *Essentials of program planning, development, management, evaluation: A manual for school speech, hearing and language programs*. Washington, D. C.: American Speech and Hearing Association.
MARTIN, E. W. (1975). "The right to education: Issues facing the speech and hearing profession," *Asha*, 17, 382-387.
MILLER, M. H., AND L. J. DEUTSCH. (1983). "Future directions in audiology," *Asha*, 25, 39-42.
MOEHLMAN, A. B. (1951). *School administration*. Cambridge, Mass: The Riverside Press.
MOLL, K. L. (1974). "Special reports, establishing professional identity: The need," *Asha*, 16, 67-68.
NEAGLEY, R. L., AND N. D. EVANS. (1970). *Handbook for effective supervision of instruction* (rev. edition). Englewood cliffs, N.J.: Prentice-Hall, Inc.
O'TOOLE, T. (1970). "Accountability and the clinician in the schools," *Language, Speech and Hearing Services in Schools*, 3, 24-25.
PENDERGAST, K. (1983). "Accountability in a public school setting," *Seminars in Speech and Language*, 4, 131-145.
PODEMSKI, R. S., B. J. PRICE, T. E. C. SMITH, AND G. E. MARSH II. (1984). *Comprehensive administration of special education*. Rockville, Md.: Aspen Systems Corp.
PUBLIC LAW 94-142, Education of All Handicapped Children Act of 1975. U. S. Government Printing.
SAXE, R. W. (1975). *School community interaction*. Berkeley, Calif.: McCutchan Publishing Corp.
———. (1965). *Speech and hearing therapy: A resource manual*. Towson, Md.: Baltimore County Public Schools.
———. (1982). *Speech, hearing and language therapy: A resource manual* (rev. edition). Towson, Md.: Baltimore County Public Schools.
TAYLOR, JOYCE S. (1980). "Public school speech-language certification standards: Are they standard?" *Asha*, 22, 159-165.
VAN HATTUM, R. J. (1965). *Clinical speech in the schools: Organization and management*. Springfield, Ill.: Charles C Thomas.
———. (1982). *Speech-language programming in the schools*. Charles C. Thomas.

6 Community-Based Speech-Language-Hearing Clinic Administration

Fred H. Bess*

INTRODUCTION

The administrator's role in the management of a community-based hearing and speech center is more far-reaching and challenging today than ever before. The field of communication disorders has undergone significant change during the past several years, and consequently, the profession lies at a significant and critical crossroad in its young and exciting history. For the past several decades, communication disorders has received substantial support from our state and federal governments, and we have been dependent upon those sources. This support, designed to improve the services to all communicatively disordered citizens and to provide a basic foundation for our profession, was readily available for educational training programs, clinical services and research. However, we have now reached a level of maturity within our profession at which we can no longer depend on government support for our existence. We now have an ample supply of speech-language pathologists and audiologists, if not too many; the concept of health care for the communicatively disordered population is now firmly imbedded into our society; and numerous universities and clinics are actively involved in research concerned with the basic and

*Dr. Bess is professor and director, Division of Hearing and Speech Sciences, Vanderbilt University School of Medicine and director, Bill Wilkerson Hearing and Speech Center, Nashville, Tennessee.

applied areas of the discipline. Stated otherwise, government has made its initial investment, and the time has come for communication disorders to "sink or swim" on its own merits.

In addition to historical factors, other important forces now impacting on the profession of communication disorders will no doubt influence our future. In the past ten years, we have witnessed dramatic changes in the way in which communicative disorders is practiced and the way in which our clinical services are delivered. Contributing to these changes have been technological developments, an increasing regulation of the entire health care industry, social change, changes in the organization of general health care delivery, shifting priorities, and changes in the mechanisms for financing health care. All of these factors are exerting a significant influence on the utilization of health care services in communication disorders, and although the precise impact of present and future developments defies definition or measurement, it is clear that a unique challenge will be presented to the discipline of communication disorders. How we respond to these developments, pressures and influences will have a significant bearing on the success of our future (Bess, 1983).

First, we must recognize that to respond effectively to change, we ourselves must change. We must reconceptualize who we are and why we are here in light of the changes that are occurring in our society. For many of us, change may be a complex and difficult process. We have invested considerable time and effort into specific philosophies and procedures, and we tend to be rather fiercely defensive about doing things in a certain way. We must learn an important lesson, however, from examples of institutions that failed to change with the changing world. The railroad industry, for example, was the largest in the U.S. economy, and not too long ago the Pennsylvania Railroad was hailed as the best-managed institution in our country. As times changed, however, and the railroads did not, they tumbled dramatically from their eminence and were rapidly outdistanced by other forms of transportation. To take another example, the American automobile industry is currently struggling desperately to catch up with changes that threaten to leave it by the side of the road.

Summarizing to this point, it should be quite evident that health care delivery in communication disorders is in a constant state of motion. Hence, today's administrator in a community-based hearing and speech setting is faced with an ever-changing profession that must be interlocked with an ever-changing society.

DESCRIPTION OF A COMMUNITY-BASED HEARING AND SPEECH CENTER

The Division of Hearing and Speech Sciences, to which this author is associated, is an autonomous division within the Vanderbilt University School of Medicine. The program is housed in, and associated with, the Bill Wilkerson Hearing and Speech Center, a large private, nonprofit, community-based corporation chartered under the laws of the State of Tennessee. The center is a multifaceted institution offering comprehensive programs in service, teaching and research. Although the division and the Bill Wilkerson Center are independent agencies, they are often looked upon as one organization, and their programs are closely coordinated in a three-fold mission, (1) to provide comprehensive, diagnostic and habilitative/rehabilitative services to individuals with communicative handicaps; (2) to conduct basic and applied research in the broad areas of communication and its disorders; and (3) to maintain an educational program designed to train future professionals in communication disorders. The underlying philosophy of the administration then is to help ensure that the center is able to achieve its maximum potential in realizing this mission.

Review of Programs

The center and division have a professional and support staff of more than sixty individuals, and a graduate enrollment of about forty students. The center receives more than 25,000 patient visits each year from residents of Tennessee and several surrounding states. The composition of the patient load represents a fairly typical mixture in a community hearing and speech center. Approximately 56 percent of the center's clients are under 15 years of age, whereas 25 percent are over 65 years. One-third of the population served would be classified as indigent.

The center provides comprehensive diagnostic and therapeutic intervention for individuals with such communicative handicaps as articulation disorders, auditory disorders, stuttering, delayed language development, hearing loss, speech impairments due to disease, stroke or accident, and voice disorders. Services are also provided for patients with swallowing disorders, cerebral palsy, developmental delays, emotional and behavioral disorders, and for the severely to profoundly handicapped. In addition, a complete hearing aid dispensary program is offered which includes hearing assessment, hearing aid selection, hearing aid purchase, and hearing aid follow-up for both individuals and groups.

An important component of the Bill Wilkerson Hearing and Speech Center is the Mama Lere Home which was founded 1966 and is located in a self-contained house immediately adjacent to the center. The purpose of the Mama Lere Home is to provide focus for parent-teaching programs in conjunction with the early identification of auditory, language, and speech deficits.

In addition to the multitude of services offered within the hearing and speech center, the staff conducts a number of outreach programs in the community. Through the rehabilitative services program, patients can be followed during the acute care stage at hospitals, to the homebound stage upon hospital discharge, and through the outpatient stage which may well involve sessions at the center. The center can thus provide an ongoing patient-clinician relationship that helps facilitate progress in patient recovery. In addition, provision of services in the home permits close interaction between the clinician and family members, and better facilitates modifications of the home environment in the patient's best interest. Patients with speech, language, or swallowing problems due to neurological or surgical causes comprise the majority of the rehabilitation services caseload. Audiological outreach services are also provided through several hospitals and private physicians' offices.

Finally, comprehensive speech, hearing, and language services are available to public and private schools.

A basic premise of the Bill Wilkerson Hearing and Speech Center is that all individuals will be admitted to the center for evaluation and treatment without respect to age, race, creed, or ability to pay. Fees are based on a sliding scale with reductions totaling about $200,000 annually.

The educational and research components of the center are operated in conjunction with Vanderbilt University. Since the educational program at Vanderbilt is housed in the center, its master's and doctoral level students are actively involved in the program. The center provides inservice training and consulting services to nurses, teachers, physicians, and other speech and hearing professionals. Consultative services in industrial noise, including hearing conservation, are also provided.

Together with its responsible teaching role, the center has a rapidly growing and diversified research program. It maintains five computer-based laboratories and each year research projects are conducted in both the applied and basic aspects of hearing, language, and speech science. The common thread that ties this diverse program together is the singular purpose of attaining new insights into the nature of communicative impairments.

Both the Division of Hearing and Speech Sciences and the Bill Wilkerson Hearing and Speech Center are self-sustaining—that is, each institution must generate sufficient revenue from its programs to provide for its levels of operations. Most of the author's comments represent a direct reflection of experiences in this environment.

Administrative Structure

An organizational scheme used at the Bill Wilkerson Hearing and Speech Center is shown in Figure 6-1. It can be seen from this chart that the director of the center also serves as the director of the Division of Hearing and Speech Sciences program at Vanderbilt University School of Medicine. The director's source of authority and responsibilty is the board of directors and the dean of the medical school. The board of directors is composed of about twenty-five community leaders interested in serving the community and the communicatively handicapped. This board serves in an advisory capacity to the director and oversees the center's operational activities. Thus, the director must interface with both members of the community and academia.

The medical director, a physician who is employed at the center on a part-time basis, is responsible for the coordination and development of medical services. Some of the responsibilities of this position include: (1) providing professional consultative services to the center; (2) offering direct medical services for patients of the center; (3) serving as a liaison between the center and the medical community; and (4) working in association with the director to maintain responsibility for third-party reimbursement and to maintain ongoing contact with state and federal agencies.

The current administrative organization of the Center is composed of the director, the academic coordinator, the coordinators for speech-language pathology

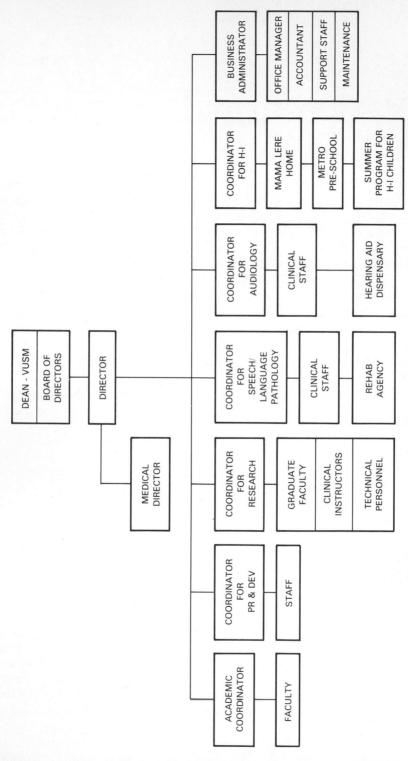

FIGURE 6-1 Organizational Scheme of the Bill Wilkerson Hearing and Speech Center.

and audiology, the coordinator for hearing-impaired children, the coordinator for public relations and development, the coordinator for research, and a business administrator. This group, along with an at-large appointed staff member, constitutes what is known as the Administrative Committee. The committee serves in an advisory capacity to the director of the center and assists the director in the development of policies and procedures affecting both the center and the division.

Sources of Support

The sources of support for the center, excluding the division budget, are summarized in Table 6-1. The data for 1977 are included and contrasted with 1984 simply to illustrate how the center has changed its funding base over a seven-year period. Not only has the overall amount increased dramatically, but there are also significant percentage changes in the various line items. Note for example, that 42 percent of the operating budget in 1977 was supported through state and/or federal funds. Most of this funding was used for service delivery programs. By 1984, the percentage of grant support was only 10 percent. Two other noticeable differences between the 1977 and 1984 budgets are the healthy increase in contributions (from $47,800 to $170,300) and the rather marked increase (from $187,500 to $622,900) in program service fees. These data illustrate the center's positive response to a need for change through improved business practices, program development, marketing, and fund raising. Each of these areas will be discussed further in the narrative to follow.

THE CHANGING ROLES OF THE ADMINISTRATOR

Management and Strategic Planning

As stated earlier, professionals in communication disorders have been very slow to change, not only in the types of services offered but in the way in which these services are administered. The story of the Bill Wilkerson Center illustrates the point rather nicely. In the 1950s and 1960s, the center experienced steady growth and development. Federal and state agencies were plentiful and generous, and the

TABLE 6-1 An Analysis of Revenue for the Bill Wilkerson Hearing and Speech Center

	1977		1984	
	AMOUNT	%	AMOUNT	%
Contributions	$ 47,800	9.7	$ 170,300	15.6
Associated Organizations	—0—	—0—	69,300	6.4
Grants	207,500	42.0	110,100	10.1
Program Service Fees	187,500	38.0	622,900	57.2
United Way	11,000	2.2	82,300	7.6
Other Revenue (Invest. & Conf.)	40,100	8.1	34,700	3.2
Total Revenue	$493,900	100.0	$1,089,600	100.0

caseload was greater than we could handle. By the mid-1970s, however, significant changes were occuring, all of which had critical impact on our organization: 1) federal and state dollars began to dwindle; 2) competition for providing speech and hearing services within the community increased tenfold; and 3) the income from fees for service declined severely. The Bill Wilkerson Center was operating no differently as an organization than it did with great success in the 1950s, but the world around us had changed dramatically. By 1977, at a time when the national economy was very poor, the future of the center was shaky. It began to appear that we did not know how to make a living as a profession, now that the state and federal governments were withdrawing support. To counter this, the center undertook a very careful analysis and assessment of every component of the agency. Following this analysis, a special task force was assembled to redesign and reshape the center's future. We began by simply restating our mission and discussing our strengths and weaknesses. We then projected the needs of the future based on the analysis of economic forecasts, projected changes in government, demographic and social changes, and competition, and we assessed how we might implement change to meet these needs. For example, we examined the cost effectiveness and cost potential of various programs with the intent of cutting some programs altogether and expanding others. We faced the fact that we could no longer be all things to all people, but instead should capitalize on our strengths, those services which we do best and which we are uniquely qualified to provide.

One area that was difficult for all of our staff involved in this process was the pricing of our services. For many years, all of us in the profession have undervalued and underpriced our services. Our clinical staff wished simply to establish a "fair price." Members of our board, however, all of whom are business people, continually proposed the question: "What price will the market bear?" In business (and health care is a business) the product is worth what the customers are willing to pay for it. The value that a patient places on our services as against competitive alternatives, depends on the patient's perception of differences in services. As Feldman (1981) has pointed out, services that come free carry a lesser value in the eyes of the consumer. The outcome of this long, hard, tedious procedure has yielded some outstanding benefits. We are now a much more efficient and cost-effective organization.

The strategic planning that leads to this outcome is the responsibility of the administrator. It is the administrator who is expected to offer the leadership, to help create the vision, and to motivate as well as facilitate key personnel to develop and implement the objectives of the center. Let us now review some of the key elements in the development of a strategic plan for the management of a community-based hearing and speech center. At a minimum, these elements include developing short- and long-term objectives, human resource strategies, and an efficient business office system.

Developing Objectives

The key personnel (i.e., the administrative committee) within any hearing and speech center need to convene regularly to discuss the policies and procedures of the institution. One of the most important tasks that this group must undertake each year is the development of short-term and long-range planning, that is, establishing the objectives of the organization. Toward this end, the agency needs to reassess on an annual basis the mission of the institution, to review strengths and weaknesses of the program and, perhaps most importantly, to assess changes that occur within our society from an economic, governmental, demographic and competitive point of view. For example, it is important to note that with the increase in the aging population, there will be an increasing prevalence of such disorders as cerebral vascular disease and neurologic conditions that are known to produce speech-language disorders. The prevalence of hearing impairment among this group is also expected to increase. After studying the impact of aging on the field of communication disorders, one can then begin to plan ways in which an organization might best take advantage of these changes. As another example, competition in our profession is on the upswing and community hearing and speech centers need to develop strategies for responding to that competition. In the 1960s and early 1970s, the Bill Wilkerson Hearing and Speech Center was the primary facility offering complete diagnostic and therapeutic services for the communicatively disordered population in mid-Tennessee. During that time period, many otolaryngologists used office staff for baseline hearing assessments, and hearing aids were purchased from hearing aid dealers. In the late 1970s otolaryngologists began to employ their own audiologists and the center realized a decrease of activity in differential diagnosis, but still remained active in the area of diagnostic evaluations, hearing aid recommendations, and therapeutic serveces. Currently, more than half the otolaryngologists in our area employ audiologists for diagnostic services, and an increasing number are dispensing amplification. With this in mind, the center moved from differential diagnosis and placed greater emphasis on the dispensing of amplification. For the past several years, we have dispensed conventional amplification systems for hearing-impaired children and adults. As a result of our long-range planning, we are also actively involved in dispensing personal FM systems now, as well as a variety of accessory devices. Furthermore, we are involved in dispensing group amplification systems to auditoriums, churches, and synagogues. We have established ourselves, prior to much of the competition, as *the* center where one should purchase amplification. The market in these areas is almost unlimited and should be pursued by all engaged in dispensing.

Once general assumptions have made within a given region, it is then possible to identify, in a realistic way, selected objectives for the center. It is important that the specific objectives established for a given year satisfy several criteria. They include:

Do the objectives match the mission of the institution?
Are we able to build on our strengths?
Do the objectives fit the assumptions that have been made?
Do they differ from business-as-usual objectives?

Once these objectives have been established, it then becomes necessary to review each objective in detail, establishing benefits, barriers and dates of implementation.

Furthermore, a plan of action needs to be established for each given objective, detailing:

Who is responsible?
How will it be accomplished?
What is the capital required?
What are the timelines?
Who is the ultimate authority?

It may be helpful to review the procedures used by the Bill Wilkerson Center administrative committee to generate planning for the past year. In essence, the committee identified twelve or thirteen different objectives that were felt to be important for the upcoming year. In order to rate these objectives, the staff was asked to assume that the goals had already been achieved and were in full operation. The objectives were then paired and the administrative committee was asked to judge which objective they thought was most important. That is, given that the center was already accomplishing two objectives very well, which one did they think was more important. All possible paired combinations were rated by the staff. In addition, the staff was asked to judge on a scale of 1-9 how well they felt they were doing with a given objective. The outcome of this analysis was then plotted on a grid such as that shown in Figure 6-2 to ascertain the group's perception of the relative importance of the various objectives. If an objective scored in the upper-left quadrant, it was considered a given, in that the staff felt that it was important, and that we were already doing quite well in achieving that objective. Those that fell in the lower-left quadrant were considered to be items of overkill—that is, we accomplish them quite well, but the managers do not feel they are very important. In the lower-right quadrant are items of discontent, those judged to be of no great value and not being accomplished very successfully either. Finally, those items that would fall into the upper-right quadrant were designated as emerging opportunities. The center was not accomplishing these objectives very well, but they were judged

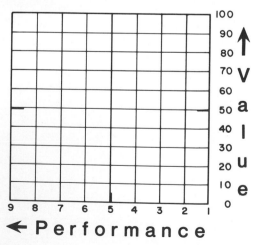

FIGURE 6-2 Graticule Used to Plot Relative Importance of Various Objectives Established from a Strategic Planning Session.

to be very important. These are the items that need a great deal of focus. Once they have been reviewed, they are then shared with the rest of the staff at the center. Each department develops a priority ranking of the objectives and in some instances adds additional items to the master list. A consensus list of objectives is then compiled and a plan of action for each objective is developed.

Human Resource Strategies

Once the objectives for the center, both short-term and long-term, have been established, it is possible to begin to develop a performance appraisal system that is consistent with the mission of the organization. That is, each department within the center can develop its own specific objectives that are in concert with the center goals. Furthermore, staff members should have the opportunity, in collaboration with their immediate supervisor, to develop their own objectives for the year, indicating how they might best assist the center in realizing its mission. In other words, we now have all of the essential ingredients for creating a performance appraisal system. It is generally agreed that such a system should result in the following: (1) a general picture of the mission of the organization; (2) a clear perception of the individual's objectives, stated in quantitative terms if possible; (3) a clear impression as to the individual's performance; (4) a general idea on how the employee might improve performance; (5) a renewed confidence in one's ability and one's general importance in the organization; (6) a clear view of how the job and objectives mesh with the individual's goals as well as the goals of the entire organization.

At this point, it is important to emphasize the role of the coordinator/manager in the performance appraisal process. The effectiveness of the process is dependent on the ability of the coordinator to conduct the evaluation in an appropriate manner. It is the coordinator who shapes the expectations and productivity of an employee; if his or her expectations are high, productivity will likewise be high. The coordinator also influences the employees' attitudes toward the job and toward themselves (Livingston, 1969).

There is no doubt that the organization as well as the employee gains from these performance appraisals. When every individual in an organization has a review of his or her responsibilities and actually has a knowledge of performance level, including needs for improvement, the organization will become stronger. It is through this individual objective planning that an organization can encourage imagination, develop individual senses of responsibility and, most importantly, intensify efforts to meet the organizational goals (Kindall and Gatza, 1963). Certainly, once the appraisal system is intact, it is much easier to administer a program using management by objectives, as well as to incorporate a system for merit.

An Efficient Business Office System

Because of the numerous changes that are occurring within the health care system, it is absolutely essential that the administrator have a firm grasp of business office practices and that he or she is able to elicit, from the business office system, appropriate information that will allow for management decisions. If an objective for the center is to develop a new intensive stuttering program, it will be important to know upstart costs, projected revenue, and an estimate of the breakeven point. Accordingly, the general purpose of a business office is to afford the director and all of the program coordinators the appropriate tools to run those programs and the center in general. These tools must be supplied on a timely and accurate basis. The best method in providing the tools to management is to have the business office systems, not the business office staff, generate the repetitive reports necessary to manage the center. The business office system must be well documented and, at a minimum, the documentation should include:

A narrative chart of accounts

A job description, detailing responsibilities and authority for each position

A description of the repetitive reports and whatever additional information is needed to input into these reports

A detailed listing as to who is authorized to perform what type of transaction

Some of the more essential reports and systems needed for the administrator to make appropriate decisions and to study the general activity of the center include the following:

SURPLUS (DEFICIT) STATEMENT FOR EACH
SEPARATE PROGRAM AS WELL AS
A COMBINED TOTAL STATEMENT

A combined balance sheet

Patient database—this should include personnel information and history of services performed

Clinician productivity reports—examples of these reports would include number of each procedure performed, revenues generated by each clinician, and/or billable hours

Accounts receivable management information—an example would include data on the aging of accounts receivable

Generation of Supplemental Income

As traditional revenue sources continue to dwindle, the administrator must seek an alternative means of income to support center programs. Two natural areas for the administrator to explore are grants and an annual giving program.

Grants Management

An essential role of the administrator is to develop appropriate skills to attract funds from foundations as well as from state and federal agencies. These funds offer a center greater flexibility for increasing staff, developing new programs, and hopefully generating additional funds in a compounding fashion. The administrator must learn to identify appropriate funding sources and then construct a competitive application using the style and format specified by the grant agency. Once a grant has been issued, there is need for continued personal contact with a project officer and the necessity of progress reports. Again, public relations is an important component to grants management.

Development of Annual Giving

It will be noted from the description of the Bill Wilkerson Center (Table 6-1) that one important source of revenue is that of gifts and contributions. This source has become increasingly important for the administrator over the past several years as federal and state dollars have continued to decrease. There are several components essential to a giving program. They include a developmental phase, an implementation phase, and a follow-up phase.

In the developmental phase of an annual giving program there is first a need to create an identity. That is, it is essential that the annual giving program have visibility within the community. At the Bill Wilkerson Center, we have developed an organization known as the Wesley Wilkerson Society, an annual giving program named after the individual who helped spearhead the development of the center. The group is composed of individuals within our community and surrounding area who contribute $1,000 or more each year. Our logo, which appropriately utilizes an ear trumpet, is shown in Figure 6-3. There is an award event each year that recognizes the members with an appropriate gift that carries the logo of the society. Hence, the concept of the Wesley Wilkerson Society is well-recognized within our community.

The second important task within the developmental phase is the hiring of a consultant. It is simply not possible for an administrator to know all of the ins and outs in the generation of a development program. Consultants are extremely valuable in identifying the appropriate prospects for solicitation, organizing and keeping records, researching all previous giving records, scheduling appointments for the

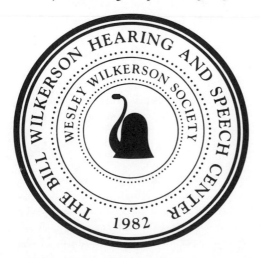

FIGURE 6-3 Logo of the Wesley Wilkerson Society — an Annual Giving Program at the Bill Wilkerson Hearing and Speech Center.

director and other key personnel with potential contributors, and ensuring that an appropriate follow-up on all prospects is made. Another feature of the developmental phase is the appointment of an advisory committee. In essence, the selection criteria for an advisory board consists of the following:

Wealth
Access to wealth
Community influence
Talent
Special relationship with agency
Work

Most important are the first two items. The specific roles of this committee are to contribute financially to the organization, assist in the identification and solicitation process, and contribute special expertise. The resources within a community for obtaining funds are many. Some of them include patients who have been helped at the center, individuals within the community, local foundations, corporations, and civil clubs and organizations. Once again, the role of public relations is quite apparent.

The next step in the development of an annual giving program is the implementation phase. This phase generally focuses on two factors: (1) development of a calendar of activities, and (2) the scheduling of appointments.

Finally, the follow-up phase involves ensuring that the donors continue to give on a regular basis. Some of the activities which can contribute to the follow-up phase are hosting a recognition award evening, revisiting with a renewal of a pledge, sending out periodic correspondence to the donors, developing special programs for giving, starting an expansion from the local community to the region, and planning for a capital funds drive.

The use of an annual giving program can be most helpful and effective for any community agency. The progress that the Bill Wilkerson Center has made over the past several years, in terms of total dollars obtained through the Wesley Wilkerson Society, is shown in Table 6-1. Note that when the program began in 1977, the center was receiving only about $48,000, but that by 1984 it was bringing in through the Wesley Wilkerson Society approximately $170,000. After an active program has been developed for several years, it is then possible to launch a capital funds drive. The Bill Wilkerson Center is now in its first such effort, with a formidable goal of $2,000,000. At this writing, the center is currently at the $1.5 million mark.

Developing and Marketing New Programs

The administrator and managing staff must recognize that because we are a dynamic profession, new programs need to be developed that ideally will satisfy three criteria: (1) the unique capabilities and expertise of the center staff; (2) the needs within the community; and (3) a minimal amount of external competition. For example, the Bill Wilkerson Hearing and Speech Center is currently in the process of developing a new day care closed Head Injury Program. After surveying the available services for this population, it became evident that there was a genuine need for a long-term day care program within the mid-Tennessee region. It was also apparent that the staff of the Bill Wilkerson Hearing and Speech Center already had much of the expertise needed to implement a successful program.

Once the decision is made to implement a new program, it is important that everything possible be done to market that program within the community. The lay public and the professional community need to be made thoroughly aware of the need of such a program and its availability within your center. There are a variety of ways in which this can be accomplished. First, the news media—radio, television and newspapers can provide you with excellent exposure and reach a large segment of the population within your community. Interest stories on patients who have benefited from the program and factual stories outlining prevalence data and need can provide valuable assistance in the launching of a new program. In addition to the use of public media, professional announcements or letters should be sent to physicians and other potential referral sources. The effective use of brochures and printed materials is also helpful. Finally, the use of advertisements for newspapers, magazines, and even television is vitally necessary as the intensity of competition in our profession increases.

Public and Customer Relations

Recall from the organization scheme (Figure 6-1) that the Bill Wilkerson Center has a coordinator for public relations and development. Such a position is vital to the character and success of an organization. In fact, enhancing the public image of the institution is an excellent marketing strategy. Reference is made to the necessity of public relations throughout this chapter. The coordinator for public relations assists the director in reaching the community with activities of the center. Presentations to various interest groups, churches, civil clubs, and professional groups, are important for the center's visibility and, in particular, for marketing new programs within the agency.

Closely allied with public relations is improving the quality of customer relations. It was once noted by Drucker (1954) that business is not determined by the producer, but by the customer. This emphasis on the customer has been universally accepted among businesses throughout the United States, but is only now beginning to surface in the field of health care delivery. One sees that numerous hospital management companies are placing a great deal of emphasis on improving customer relations in order simply to maintain their piece of the marketplace. That is, competition is becoming very keen among hospitals, private practices, and nonprofit organizations. Consequently, greater efforts are being directed at the customer or, in our instance, the patient, simply as a means of retaining those who are already coming to the institution. We should never forget that it is the customer/patient who represents our largest referral source. Thus, it is important that the administrator make efforts to ensure that staff within the center do everything possible to maintain quality guest relations. Some of the key elements in this regard include training the staff to greet patients promptly, using words that express respect and understanding, offering assistance to patients who appear to be in need, being informed and prepared, requesting and giving information clearly and concisely, and promoting pride in the staff group and the organization. Quality and/or public relations is just as important when talking on the phone or when caring for a hostile or depressed patient as it is under ordinary circumstances. Finally, the administrator can encourage the concept of quality relations by reinforcing appropriate behavior promptly and in a positive way. In the development of a program concerned with customer relations, there are a number of areas that probably should be considered. These include:

1. Communication. How can we communicate caring and understanding? How do we deal with the angry client?

2. Development of customer relations norms. Develop a list of behaviors that will become the norm in dealing with customers. These should include how you answer the phone, how clients are greeted, and client waiting facilities.

3. Barriers to customer relations. What in our organization prevents us from being customer oriented?

4. Operations analysis. This involves looking at the organization's policies and standard operating procedures to see if they are supportive or inhibitive of a customer relations approach. How can they be changed?

5. Monitoring system, customer surveys, recognition system, and performance appraisal. All are ways in which to reinforce the importance of a customer relations program.

Interfacing with Local, State and Federal Agencies

By now it should be apparent that a principal responsibility of the center director is to relate and communicate with numerous lay and professional leaders, as well as with a variety of organizations. Local affiliations are needed with, for example, physicians, educators, psychologists, social workers and counselors. Liaisons must also be developed with civic and social clubs, United Way, and health care facilities such as hospitals, home health care centers and health maintenance organizations (Rosen, 1963).

It is equally important for the administrator to interface with state and federal agencies, especially those responsible for coordinating health education and welfare. Contact is also needed for third party reimbursement agencies including insurance programs, rehabilitation services administration, and crippled childrens' services. These agencies can afford assistance not only in helping a needy patient, but many can assist the administrator in identifying funding sources for clinical programs.

SUGGESTIONS TO FUTURE SPEECH-LANGUAGE-HEARING ADMINISTRATORS IN A COMMUNITY-BASED FACILITY

It is almost superfluous to note that the average speech-language pathologist and/or audiologist receives limited training, if any, for an administrative position, and is thus poorly equipped to go into an administrator's role. Such general areas as finance, organization, marketing, public relations, fund raising, and grant writing represent the bulk of the administrator's responsibility. To date, however, there are no programs in our profession which offer courses in these areas. The aspiring administrator who wishes to work in a community-based facility needs to diversify his or her educational base, and ideally should take a minor in either business or health care administration. An educational background in health care management, managerial finance, marketing management, human resources management, and organization design would be invaluable to an administrator working in a community hearing and speech center.

Also of value would be an externship or internship in a similar facility, under the direction of a director or administrator. Perhaps as a summer experience, the individual could work as an assistant to a director in learning some of the basic responsibilities that are expected of an administrator in a major community hearing and speech center.

Finally, tomorrow's administrator must be willing to accept change—a continuing modification of our practice as changes in the environment occur. In this rapidly growing world we cannot stand still. If we are not moving ahead into the future, or at least keeping abreast of what is happening around us, we are stepping back into the past and are in danger of extinction.

SUMMARY AND CONCLUSIONS

The roles of the administrator in a community hearing and speech center are many, and require skills far beyond what is taught in traditional programs in communication disorders. The greatest challenges focus on finances and competition. The administrator must develop a sound business system that will allow for intelligent management decisions and explore all possible avenues for generating funds, while at the same time warding off increasing competition. It is a position that requires decisiveness, flexibility, some imagination, considerable skill in personal relations, and much patience. It is a formidable task indeed, but one which offers, in addition to challenge, a satisfying and fulfilling professional career.

REFERENCES

BESS, F. H. (July 1983). "Critical issues in clinical audiology." Paper presented at the Western Regional Conference, American Speech-Language-Hearing Association, Honolulu.
DRUCKER, P. (1954). *The practice of management*. New York: Harper and Row.
FELDMAN, A. S. (December 1981). "The challenge of autonomy," *Asha*, 941–945.
KINDALL, A. F. AND J. GATZA. (November-December 1963). "Positive program for performance appraisal," *Harvard Business Review*, 153–160.
LIVINGSTON, J. S. (1969). "Pygmalion in management," *Harvard Business Review*, July-August, 81–89.
ROSEN, J. (1961). "The community speech and hearing center as a representative of the profession," *Asha*, 3, 117–119.

7 Administration of Community Hospital Speech-Language-Hearing Programs

Twila Strandberg Griffith*

INTRODUCTION

The speech-language pathologist or audiologist who develops and directs a hospital-based service faces a dual challenge. The first is to know the business of health care. The second is to acquire and practice sound principles of management. Each requires continuous study and effort. Management is not a do-it-yourself task. Some additional, formal training in the basic management skills is needed by most of us (Drucker, 1974).

It is the purpose of the hospital speech-language pathology and audiology program to provide comprehensive professional services in the evaluation and treatment of communication disorders. This purpose is served when there are clear goals and objectives established and effective procedures designed to meet them—all under the leadership and management of the experienced speech-language pathologist or audiologist.

This chapter is not intended as a "how-to" approach to managing a hospital service. Rather, it identifies some of the management areas, large and small, that must be addressed in the conduct of a vaiable service.

---

*Dr. Griffith is director, Speech, Language and Hearing Services, Sarah Bush Lincoln Health Center, Mattoon, Illinois.

Hospitals

In the past decade, there has been a slow, steady increase in the number of speech-language pathology and audiology services in hospitals, long-term care facilities and home health agencies. This chapter will describe the organization and management of speech and hearing services in the health care setting with primary emphasis on services in community hospitals. The American Hospital Association (AHA) defines a community hospital as a nonfederal, short-term general or other special hospital whose facilities and services are available to the public (American Hospital Association Hospital Statistics, 1985). Community hospitals vary in size from less than 100 beds to more than 500 beds and are located in both urban and rural settings. Speech and hearing services are available to both inpatients and outpatients and, are, in many instances, provided on a consultancy basis to other types of health care facilities and agencies.

The emphasis on community hospitals is made with good reason as they employ a rapidly growing segment of our profession. In 1974, 6,549 hospitals responded on the annual survey of the AHA (Hospital Statistics, 1974). Of this sample, 1,387 (21.2%) reported speech therapy services. Of the hospitals responding 5,412 were classified as general and other special hospitals and 996 of that subgroup (18.4%) offered speech therapy services. One decade later in 1984, of 6,353 hospitals responding 5,400 were general and other special hospitals and 2,175 (40.3%) reported speech pathology services.

Strandberg (1974) surveyed 1,209 of the 1,387 member hospitals reporting speech services on the AHA annual survey. She found that the largest number of speech-language pathology services were in nongovernment, not-for-profit hospitals. Over 90% of these services were in general or other special hospitals. While it was not the principal concern of her study, some data were obtained concerning audiology services. Fifty-nine percent of the hospitals surveyed reported that they employed between one and four audiologists, either full or part time. The number of hospitals offering only audiology services was not determined. The AHA does not include audiology as a service on their annual survey. This is surprising since, historically, audiology services were thought to be present in many hospitals having no speech-language service. Speech-language pathology and audiology services in federal government hospitals, for example, Veterans' Administration hospitals, are well known. However, the proportion of this type of hospital is small.

The community hospital, contrasted with a special service facility such as a children's hospital, is open to the public for all types of services. A community hospital speech and hearing service is likely to relate directly to other health care settings. These would include long-term care facilities and home health agencies.

Long-Term Care

Speech and hearing services are provided to a limited extent in long-term care facilities. *Nursing Home, Extended Care Facility, Geriatric Center,* and *Home for the Aged* are all names for long-term care facilities, and can mean different things in different places (Griffith and Strandberg, 1982). These names are confusing because there is no standard classification system. The name may reflect the facility's philosophy of care, the kind of service provided or the type of resident accepted. One classification system is based on the source of payment for the residents' care. This includes skilled nursing facilities and intermediate care facilities. This classification is helpful to the speech and hearing professional in understanding the types of services and methods of reimbursement.

A *skilled nursing facility* (SNF) provides skilled nursing care and other services under professional direction with frequent medical supervision. Such facilities are for residents who need the type of care and treatment required during the post-acute phase of illness or during recurrence of symptoms in long-term illness. A wide range of specialized medical and rehabilitation services.

An *intermediate care facility* (ICF) provides basic nursing care and other restorative services under periodic medical direction. Such facilities are for residents who have long-term illnesses or disabilities which may have reached a relatively stable condition.

Most states license *intermediate care facilities for the developmentally disabled.* In these facilities, an attempt is made to provide an environment that closely resembles the everyday world so these persons can learn independence and can interact with the community. In some areas there may be another type of long-term care facility called *sheltered care* which provides personal assistance, supervision and suitable activities. There are alternatives to long-term care. Adult *day care* and *respite care* make it possible for the patient to remain at home for a longer period.

Home Health Services

A home health agency may be a public or private agency that provides skilled nursing care and other rehabilitation services in the home. It may be part of a hospital program or a separate organization. Home health services may be organized under the Visiting Nurse Association, private, not-for-profit agencies or government agencies, to serve a specified region. Qualified agencies may provide services for Medicare and/or Medicaid patients including skilled nursing care, physical therapy, occupational therapy, speech-language pathology, social services and home health aid or homemaker services to homebound patients.

Accreditation, Certification and Licensure

The Joint Commission on Accreditation of Hospitals (JCAH) establishes standards for the operation of hospitals and other health-related facilities. These standards are published annually in an accreditation manual. The 1986 edition of the Accreditation Manual for Hospitals (AMH/86) (1985) contains new standards which became effective July 1, 1986. These revised standards resulted from regulations developed by the Health Care Financing Administration (HCFA) which exempted certain hospital rehabilitation programs from the Medicare prospective payment system (PPS) (Downey, White and Karr, 1984). The AMN/86 outlines the standards for rehabilitation hospitals and for comprehensive rehabilitation units within acute care hospitals. The impact of the 1986 standards on speech-language pathologist and audiologists is fully explained by White (1986). All departments in hospitals that seek accreditation must meet these standards.

Two additional accrediting groups for speech-language pathology and audiology services are the Council on Accreditation of Rehabilitation Facilities (CARF) and the Professional Services Board (PSB) of the American Speech-Language-Hearing Association (ASHA).

While accreditation is the term used for the evaluation process performed by a private organization, government agencies follow a certification process to evaluate an institution that meets predetermined standards. Certification is distinguished from licensure in that the lack of certification does not prevent the right to practice while licensure is a prerequisite to practice.

Different types of health care facilities are subject to different standards, rules and regulations determined and administered by government agencies and accrediting groups. Furthermore, they differ from state to state for the same settings. The reader must take the responsibility for identifying applicable standards and regulations for his or her particular setting.

In the pages to follow, the organizational and management principles and practices that apply to a community hospital speech and hearing service are presented in detail. It is reasonable to assume that many of them apply to other health care settings as well.

ADMINISTRATIVE ORGANIZATION

The components of every organization, including hospitals, are arranged according to lines of authority. Most community hospitals have a governing body referred to as *the board*. The board delegates its authority to the administrator. This administrator will have associate or assistant administrators to organize and manage various activities of the entire hospital system. There are four major types of functions: (a) nursing services, (b) fiscal services, (c) ancillary professional services, and (d) support services. Departments are designated within each of the functional groups. These departments represent "middle management" (Rowland, 1984).

The organization can be illustrated graphically in a chart which shows the basic relationships among components. The major goals and objectives are defined in the administrative policies and procedures manual. All components of the organization are governed by this manual.

The manager of Speech and Hearing Services must understand the goals and objectives established by administration, and coordinate the department with the overall plan for the hospital. A chart should show the lines of authority within the department. These lines of communication must be clearly understood by all personnel. A manual must be developed which defines the philosophy and organization of the department, states goals and objectives and describes policies and procedures. This manual is revised annually.

Department Identity

Our profession has worked diligently over the years to establish autonomy and status. This author takes the position that the community hospital Speech and Hearing Services should reflect its professional status in terms of its placement in the organization structure. In other words, Speech and Hearing Services should be independent and freestanding with department level status managed by either a certified speech-language pathologist or an audiologist. There should be some provision for autonomy of the Speech and Hearing service in the department of Physical Medicine.

The name of the service should be one that most patients can identify. Although the professional should retain the title *speech-language pathologist* or *audiologist*, the department or services may be more simply named; for example, Speech and Hearing Services. Longer names are difficult for people to remember and to read on signs. A short and easily identified name is also more effective for marketing strategies. The experienced manager does not expect the hospital administration to run the department. Speech-language pathologists and audiologists are experts in their fields and should assume responsibility for the day-to-day operation and for long-range planning.

The majority of hospital speech-language services are independent departments or located in a department of Physical Medicine and Rehabilitation managed by a physiatrist or physical therapist. Most audiology services are associated with departments of Neurology or Otolaryngology if not coordinated with Speech-Language Services in an independent department. When speech-language pathologists and audiologists work in other departments such as Physical Medicine, Otolaryngology, Neurology or Pediatrics, professional identification and autonomy are often lost.

Many speech-language services consist of one person. The administrator may know little about our field and will assume that all speech-language pathologists and audiologists are prepared to provide the administrative direction for the service. This may be difficult for those individuals whose past clinical and management experience and exposure to health care environments are limited. If there is only one position in speech-language pathology, that person will be expected to provide administration with all of the information needed to deliver speech-language services regardless of the organization level of the service.

If the organization includes an assistant director, this person assumes more administrative duties and may continue to have clinical supervisory duties in his or her certified area. An assistant director position may include responsibility for both office and professional staff, including other supervisors. The assistant director is in charge of the department in the absence of the director.

If the department organization includes clinical supervisory positions, in addition to clinical and supervisory duties, other responsibilities may include: (a) assisting in orienting and evaluating personnel, (b) maintaining productivity statistics, and (c) helping with budget preparation.

Job Descriptions

There is little consistency in the format and content of job descriptions. Some facilities specify the personal requirements necessary to perform the job, such as education, training and experience, as well as the duties to be performed. Job descriptions will vary depending upon the size of the department and type of position involved, and they range from being very specific to very general. The description must accurately reflect the responsibilities of the position so the staff person can agree to meet them, and the manager can evaluate performance accordingly. A separate job description is needed for every position, including graduate interns. All job descriptions must be reviewed annually.

Department Policies and Procedures

Planning is an important management function and policies are necessary plans. They provide broad guidelines to assist in decision making and help the staff stay within certain limits.

Procedures are also plans used to meet the objectives of the department. Procedures are more specific than policies because they must be a guide to action rather than a guide to thinking (Haimann, 1973). Procedures must describe the sequence in which the task should be performed. Speech-language pathologists and audiologists are skilled individuals who can be depended upon to develop their own sequence of activities to meet a specific objective. Therefore, procedures affecting only Speech and Hearing Services can be somewhat more general. On the other hand, if a policy and its subsequent procedures originate in Speech and Hearing but involve other departments, they must be more detailed.

A rule is different from a policy or procedure. A rules does not specify any order of conformity. For example, there may be a "no smoking" rule. There are no steps or levels involved in following this rule. It is simply followed and enforced. At times, a department manager may set up rules or enforce rules set up by the administration.

Patient Scheduling

Patients are routinely scheduled Monday through Friday. Arrangements are made to see patients on weekends when necessary. The receptionist takes the responsibility for scheduling and must be well-informed about the time needed for various procedures. All scheduling is done at the convenience of the patient. Some outpatients have restrictions such as available transportation, the need for rest time during the day, or other scheduled rehabilitation sessions. Treatment is also scheduled during the time of day when maximum performance is expected. If the patient is being seen by other services, the treatment times are coordinated.

A distinction is usually made between those patients seen only for evaluation and those who are series patients, that is, they are seen regularly over a period of weeks or months. Series patients are seen mostly by the speech-language pathologist.

An attempt is made to schedule treatments at the same time on the same days each week, with the treatment days spaced for maximum benefit. Audiology typically sees patients only for an evaluation with the exception of hearing aid evaluations. The professional staff stay on schedule so that the patient does not have to wait. More than one staff member should be familiar with each case so that treatment need not be cancelled because of illness or vacations. Treatment sessions may be rescheduled before or after a holiday but cancellations should be avoided. Most outpatient services in health care facilities are closed for seven or eight holidays during the year. In general, schedule changes should be kept to a minimum.

Sessions are scheduled for the amount of time needed for effective treatment. Inpatient sessions and those for young children may be for 30 minutes. Outpatients usually benefit from 45–60 minutes of treatment, depending on their number of sessions each week. Evaluations are scheduled for the length of time needed to complete the tests and obtain background information. The time needed for audiological procedures varies. The important point in all instances is to schedule the patient for the amount of time needed at the most convenient time for them.

Supervision of Staff

Speech-language pathologists and audiologists are competent individuals who are usually self-starters; they usually require only general supervision and they function well independently. When new or unexpected situations arise, it is helpful if the director consults with the staff concerning the nature of the problem and the possible options for its solution. This interaction helps the manager to know his or her staff and to recognize individuals who have potential for future supervisory or management responsibilities. Staff members who have no prior experience in health care appreciate supervision.

A staff member in the Clinical Fellowship Year is supervised according to the requirements of the American Speech-Language-Hearing Association. As they learn the requirements of the hospital, they become more confident. In some cases it is necessary to be more directive regarding their ability to function independently, for they may be capable of doing more than they realize. Most graduate interns will work under very close supervision. In some situations, it is essential to have staff members with the interns at all times.

The most important aspect of managing people is to be consistent from day to day and from person to person. The staff should have clear policies and detailed procedures to guide them, and supervision that is readily available to support and assist them.

Performance Evaluations

An important aspect of staff management is the annual performance evaluation. Both the manager and the staff member should prepare well for these evaluations and schedule a time when there will be no interruptions. During the evaluation, accomplishments can be measured against performance standards. New goals can then be set. Poor performance or unacceptable behavior should not be ignored or allowed to continue until evaluation time. Small problems should be taken care of immediately or they may become large ones.

Staff

The strongest speech and hearing departments are autonomous and self-supporting, which means they operate entirely on revenues generated by the professional staff. While it is important to maintain productivity goals, the major concern of the service should be the quality of care provided to the patient. ASHA suggests that professional personnel have no less than 15 percent of their work week designated to develop treatment plans, write reports, complete discharge plans and participate in patient staffings (ASHA, PSB Standards, 1980). This sets the maximum load for any speech-language pathologist or audiologist at six hours of patient care per day. It is difficult to make general statements regarding staffing needs. Effective managers will consider the following: that (a) schedules and resources are arranged as conveniently as possible, (b) appropriate materials and equipment are conveniently located, and (c) their time should be used evaluating and treating patients rather than writing notes by hand, filing charts and developing treatment materials. It is reasonable to assume that one hour of treatment requires 2.1 to 2.5 manhours.

Space and Location

The AMH/86 (1985) requires that each rehabilitation department have adequate space, facilities and equipment to fulfill professional, educational and administrative needs (p.222). Since space is extremely expensive, assigned space must be well utilized and requests for additional space carefully justified. The reception area should be attractive, well furnished and orderly. Chairs must be comfortable with arms that provide support for hemiplegic patients. A children's table and chairs should be available. Current magazines and coffee are welcome courtesies.

Ideally, the department should be near an outside entrance. Adequate parking, all doors, restroom facilities, elevators, telephones and drinking fountains should be easily accessible to wheelchair patients. Attractive signs that are easily read and understood are essential. Speech and Hearing Services should be close to other rehabilitation services, particularly physical therapy and occupational therapy.

It goes without saying that Speech and Hearing Services should be located in a quiet area. Carpeting keeps the noise down, especially if it is installed on both the walls and floors. In audiology, this is particularly effective. Treatment rooms should be comfortable for children and adults. If the majority of the patients are adults, the supplies and decorations for children should be kept out of sight so the room looks appropriate to adults.

Equipment and Materials

Equipment and materials adequate to meet the needs of the professional and support staff are a management responsibility. Equipment must be of a type, quality and quantity designed to provide safe and effective patient care (AMH/86

p. 223). Poorly functioning equipment and inadequate materials result in reduced productivity and quality of care. Office machines require regular maintenance and replacement at appropriate intervals. The manager must establish a clear procedure for acquisition of office supplies and a method of maintaining inventories.

Speech-Language Services

Many departments separate staff office space from evaluation/treatment rooms. In reality, it works very well to have each speech-language pathologist in a comfortable combined office/treatment area equipped so the pathologist can use it for evaluation and treatment of both adults and children. The furniture should be of good quality, comfortable, and in good repair. Some state departments of health require hand-washing facilities in any room designated as a treatment area. All surfaces in the room, especially the treatment table, should be covered with a material such as formica that can be sprayed with a germicidal product. Wood surfaces may not meet Public Health standards. Chairs used in the treatment room should be comfortable and have arms. The height and leg space under the treatment table must be appropriate for use by patients in wheelchairs.

A materials center that is conveniently located, well lighted and has sufficient drawer and shelf space is essential. Each speech-language pathologist should have a cassette tape recorder and a small dictating unit. In addition to the materials used to evaluate and treat communication disorders, it is important to include adult materials for teaching reading, writing and numerical skills. Duplicate sets of all frequently used items are a convenience for a large staff with members who travel.

Audiology Services

Rooms utilized by the audiologists should be in a quiet, low-traffic area and accessible to both wheelchair and gurney. Equipment for a basic hospital-based audiology service includes: (a) a soundproof booth large enough to accommodate patients in wheelchairs; (b) a two-channel diagnostic audiometer, soundfield amplifier and two speakers; (c) a diagnostic impedance/otoadmittance bridge or meter (not screening); (d) visual reinforcement audiometry (VRA) with lighted toys; (e) stereo tape deck and test tapes; (f) otoscope(s); and (g) calibration equipment or arrangements for calibration.

If an industrial hearing conservation program is to be developed, additional equipment may be needed such as a (a) sound level meter and/or dosimeter; (b) selection of ear protectors; (c) portable pure-tone audiometer; and (d) small industrial screening booth to free the large booth for clinical use.

A service which does not wish to dispense, but plans to do hearing aid evaluations and make earmolds will need additional equipment including a wide selection of clinic or test hearing aids, a selection of stock earmolds of different sizes and types, earmold tubing, earhooks and batteries.

Actual hearing aid dispensing requires considerably more basic equipment.

Financial arrangements and accounts must be established for hearing aid purchase from the manufacturers. A detailed description of the needs for preparing a dispensing service is provided in Loavenbruck and Madell (1981).

The purchase of electronystagmography (ENG) and brainstem evoked response (BSER) equipment involves several considerations, including cost, space restrictions, and needs of the medical staff (intraoperative monitoring, visual evoked potentials, somatosensory evoked potentials, 2-channel ENG recording, and so on). Sample equipment can be seen at professional conference exhibits and by arrangement with an area equipment supplier. Some companies permit the use of a "loaner" ENG or BSER unit prior to purchase. Most suppliers and manufacturers provide basic training in the use of the equipment. However, advanced training at workshops and conferences is usually necessary and these costs should be budgeted accordingly.

Inservice and Continuing Education

The department manager is responsible for meeting the inservice and continuing professional education needs of the staff. New personnel must be thoroughly oriented to the department and to the total hospital. The department budget should include funds for staff professional education away from the facility, such as annual conferences, workshops and seminars. There is value in arranging for the staff to present inservice programs as well as attend them. Professional reference materials can be obtained in the medical library. Professional books, journals and a reprint file are helpful.

Monitoring the Quality of Care

The quality assurance program is very important to patient care and for standards compliance. In most hospitals, the authority for the quality assurance (or comprehensive care) program comes from the administration and hospital board and is included in the by-laws of the medical staff. All rehabilitation services are responsible for a planned and systematic procedure to determine and monitor the quality of care provided to the patient. In addition, it is necessary to specify how problems documented in a review have been resolved.

Data Collection

Systematic data collection concerning all aspects of departmental operations and activities is another important management function. These data are necessary for developing budgets, staffing plans and marketing programs. The responsibilities for recording and reporting department statistics can be shared among the director, supervisors and secretarial staff. The hospital accounting department can offer guidelines for recording and summarizing these data. The basic types of data that might be collected monthly are:

SPEECH-LANGUAGE PATHOLOGY

Activity and Revenue for:
1. Inpatients
   a. Medicare Inpatients
   b. Inpatient Treatment Hours
2. Outpatients
   a. Outpatient Treatment Hours
   b. Homebound Patients
   c. Homebound Treatment Hours
3. Consultancy Services
   a. Billable Services

AUDIOLOGY

Activity and Revenue for:
1. Inpatients
   a. Number of each procedure by type and time
2. Outpatients
   a. Number of each procedure by type and time
3. Number of Industrial Audiograms
4. Number of Hearing Aids Dispensed
5. Staff Productivity

Departmental statistics for patient care are submitted monthly to prepare the monthly operating report (MOR) for the department. The MOR shows the month's activities in terms of patients seen, hours of treatment provided or procedures completed, revenues, and expenses for the month. These data are compared for actual and budgeted amounts. Prior months and the previous year's totals may also be included for review. The department's contribution margin, that is, ratio of revenue to expense, is indicated. The MOR provides a continuous study of department activity and productivity.

Records and Documentation

The need for accountability cannot be overemphasized. Documentation must be thorough and must follow the regulations of the setting in which treatment is provided. A comprehensive rehabilitation record should include: reason for referral; summary of the clinical condition; evaluation; plan of treatment with measurable goals; and progress notes. As treatment continues, the monthly summaries can discuss the patient and/or the family's attitude regarding treatment, results of additional assessments, justification for continued treatment and expected improvement in functional ability. Recommendations for further care must be included in the discharge summary.

PROBLEM-ORIENTED MEDICAL RECORDS

Documentation procedures in hospitals and other health care settings are subject to rules and regulations. Bouchard and Shane (1977) found little consistency among speech-language pathologists in their documentation and recording methods. They suggest the use of the Problem-Oriented Medical Record (POMR), which was designed specifically for medical record keeping, as one approach to establishing some consistency for speech-language pathologists and audiologists. A component of the POMR is the SOAP format used to address each problem listed on the record. SOAP is an acronym for Subjective, Objective, Assessment and Plan, the four categories used to separate information on the patient's record.

Uses of the POMR and "soaping" for speech-language pathologists and audiologists are also described by Balich et al. (1978).

CHARTING PROCEDURES

There are some basic procedures used universally for making entries in the patient's chart. Every inpatient visit is immediately charted noting the service, the date and the time. Military time may be required. The information must be accurate, concise and legibly written in black ink. An appropriate signature completes the entry. For speech and hearing professionals this usually involves signature, title and certification:

Twila E. Griffith, Ph.D.
Speech-Language Pathologist/CCC

If regulations permit, it may be possible to use the name and SLP/CCC only for subsequent entries on the same page following the complete first entry.

Outpatient progress notes and reports may be dictated using the small dictating units. The secretary then types and files them after they are signed or initialed by the professional. For outpatient progress notes, only initials (teg) are required for subsequent entries on a page after the first entry is signed off as above.

Forms that go into the medical record must be uniform. Medical Records and/or a forms committee make the final decisions on proposed new forms. NCR forms are not recommended and special arrangements must be made before they are adopted.

OUTPATIENT RECORDS

An individual record that is complete, accurate and current must be maintained for each outpatient. An accrediting group may specify storage of all outpatient records in Medical Records rather than in the department. This assures an efficient and protected system. In this case, a procedure must be developed for retrieval of records for daily use in the department.

Outpatient records include (a) a written referral, (b) medical and other clinical information, (c) the evaluation and treatment plan, (d) progress notes for each patient visit, (e) interim treatment summaries, and (f) recertification and other authorizations required for third party payors. The treatment summaries include (a) a summary of the treatment; (b) responses of the patient; (c) current status of the problem; and (d) recommended modifications of the treatment plan. A discharge summary is prepared for each patient. A signed and dated release of information is retained in the record any time information is requested. Outpatient records are retained for twenty-five years.

Referrals

The need for a physician referral for inpatient and outpatient services is established by the State Department of Public Health, which licenses the hospital, and the Joint Commission on Accreditation of Hospitals. The AMH/86 stipulates that rehabilitation services may be initiated by qualified individuals. In general all speech-language pathology and audiology inpatient services are ordered by a staff physician. In some states the licensing act may require a physician's order for outpatient services. Third party reimbursement for outpatient services may also require a physician's order. Directors are advised to investigate their state's hospital licensing act for variations in the rules for referrals, in terms of both receiving and making them.

Ancillary Services, Allied Health and Rehabilitation Services

Speech-language pathology and audiology services are frequently classified as *ancillary services*. In a hospital, *ancillary* means a service that assists the physician in diagnosis or treatment. The term also designates a hospital department that can charge the patient directly and generate hospital revenue.

Another classification is *allied health service.* Many people wrongly assume that speech-language pathologists and audiologists are allied health professionals especially since physical therapists and occupational therapists are included in this category. There are twenty-three health occupations which collaborate with twenty-seven national medical specialty societies and the American Medical Association (AMA) to make up the Committee on Allied Health Education and Accreditation (AMA, Allied Health Education Directory, 1978). Since speech-language pathology and audiology prefer to have the American Speech-Language Hearing Association and its members make decisions regarding education and accreditation, they are not correctly classified as allied health professionals. Many individuals use this term for anyone connected with health care rather than the more accurate "health care professional."

The JCAH defines Rehabilitation Services as "all Professional and technical services that assist physically disabled persons to attain and/or retain their functional capacity."

Further, the JCAH includes speech-language pathology and audiology under *Rehabilitation Services.* The AMH/86 has expanded its description of speech, language and hearing program to include "a continuum of services, including prevention, identification, diagnosis, consultation, and the treatment of patients regarding speech, language, oral and pharyngeal sensorimotor function, hearing and balance. (AMH/86, p. 320). It is expected that the AHM/87 will contain mention of evoked potential response equipment (White, 1986).

Each individual providing rehabilitation services must "meet all applicable licensure, certification, or registration requirements" (AMH/86, p. 222). If the organization of the hospital includes a Director of Rehabilitation or Physical Medicine, the Speech and Hearing Services will probably not have department level status. In a separate autonomous service, the speech-language pathology or audiology director assumes responsibility for the total function of the department and reports directly to one of the hospital administrators.

Departments of Physical Medicine usually have a physician as medical director. A physician-member of the medical staff who is knowledgeable in a rehabilitation service may act as the medical liaison for rehabilitation services. It is strongly recommended that the patient's primary physician retains responsibility if the patient is referred for rehabilitation services. If this is not possible, the physician directing or supervising rehabilitation may assume responsibility. The program should be coordinated with the primary care physician to provide continuity of care. Separate rehabilitation services respond effectively to a medical staff committee appointed annually by the chief of the medical staff. Ideally, the committee should be composed of specialists from Family Practice, Neurology, Otolaryngology, Pediatrics, Internal Medicine, and Orthopedics. In this situation, each rehabilitation service is free to relate directly to the physician who is primarily responsible for the patient and to all other medical staff members as needed.

FINANCIAL MANAGEMENT

The Budget Process

The fiscal management of hospitals has become increasingly complex. The change from what once was a comparatively simple bookkeeping function to very complicated financial management has been dictated by the government (Beck, 1980). Speech-language pathologists and audiologists frequently need both insight and instruction regarding their budgetary responsibilities. Fortunately, hospitals have fiscal officers and specialists in all budgetary processes to work with the department managers. It is not possible to have a workable budget without department input.

The Capital Budget

Department capital budget projections are often requested prior to completion of the annual budget. The capital budget concerns the purchase of new equipment. There may be two kinds of capital budget projections requested, those for the current year and those for long-range planning. Three- to five-year capital expenditure projections for items expected to exceed a specified dollar amount are forwarded to Fiscal Services and are used to make up a tentative budget. The actual expenditures are not approved at this stage. They must be resubmitted for approval in the quarter in which the equipment is to be purchased.

The current year's budget will include all of the department's capital needs regardless of the amount. The manager ranks them in order of importance and identifies each as an addition, a replacement or an improvement. The manager is usually required to write a brief description of the item and discuss how it will support the goals of the department and the hospital.

The Annual Operating Budget

Regardless of the type of budget process used, the process begins with a budget calendar which gives timelines for each part. Fiscal Services acts as a resource to support the manager's budgeting plans. The controller directs the overall budget process and assists in the development of reasonable projections of departmental activities. There is no substitute for the manager's thorough knowledge of the financial parameters of the department's operation. Further, the manager's professional expertise and judgment should prevail in budgetary decisions that affect the delivery of care.

Budget projections are based on historical data from department statistics and data provided by Fiscal Services. The reasons for variances in the current budget need to be identified to prevent their recurrence. Projections are made in each of the areas that follow:

Department Activity

Department activity can be expressed in several ways such as number of treatment hours or number of procedures and time of each procedure. In making projections, it is helpful to (a) observe changes in activity, study their causes and determine if they represent trends that will continue; (b) anticipate changes in patient flow; (c) consider the impact of new services and/or equipment; and (d) consider changes in standards of care, medical staff, or management philosophy. The director must then make projections for inpatient services, outpatient services, and special activities for the next budget year.

Productivity and Staffing

Productivity for speech-language services can be stated in terms of worked manhours per treatment hour. For audiology, time per procedure must be calculated and converted to treatment hours. A productivity goal is a necessity in determining all staffing needs. Factors to consider in determining this goal are (a) observed changes from year-to-year, their causes and possible trends; (b) achievement of the previous year's productivity goals; (c) anticipated changes that would affect the staffing patterns; (d) impact of new services and equipment; (e) changes in standards or management philosophy that will affect staffing; and (f) decisions regarding modification of the pay scale.

Revenue Parameters

When looking at the revenue projections for the budgetary process, consider (a) any change in the unit by which revenue is measured; (b) whether increased patient flow can be handled with the present staff and improved productivity;

(c) if present charges will cover inflationary or deflationary impact; and (d) any cost trends, changes in case/service mix or charge structures which may occur before the beginning of the next fiscal year.

Expense Parameters

Estimates of departmental expenses must consider every item of expenditure including wages and salaries, fringe benefits, minor equipment purchases, educational activities, travel, and supplies. A unit of measure is selected for each expense to show how it is distributed over the budget year, e.g., monthly or semiannually. These factors should be considered (a) if the unit of measure adopted is appropriate for the type of expense incurred; (b) if trends and their causes other than inflation are identified; and (c) if any unanticipated new costs arise, such as maintenance contracts for equipment on which the "free service warranty" has expired.

After all of the projections have been completed, it must be determined if the projected departmental activity will create enough revenue to cover the projected expense parameters. For a department to be self-supporting and independent, the revenues must completely pay for the service and, in addition, contribute a profit margin to help pay for the departments that are not fee-based.

Fiscal Services reviews the projections from all departments and compiles them into a preliminary budget. A meeting is then arranged in which the manager discusses the budget with an administrator and representatives from Fiscal Services. After review and approval by the board and administrators, the department operating budgets are finalized for distribution to the department managers.

Wage and Salary Scale

Since a significant portion of the department expense is wages and salaries, it is important to understand how these are determined and applied to speech-language pathologists and audiologists. Rowland (1984) states that most hospitals approach wages and salaries in the same way. After a job analysis is completed and a job description developed, pertinent information about the specific nature of the job is collected. Following the data collection, information is obtained regarding the salaries of comparable jobs in the community and surrounding area. The current job market and cost-of-living also furnish guidelines.

Benefits

Benefits typically include paid vacation, sick and holiday time, and some form of health insurance coverage. The health insurance plan may include hospitalization, outpatient services, and vision and dental care. Life insurance, long-term disability insurance and accident insurance are also significant benefits. Discounts at the cafeteria and pharmacy and free parking are appealing to the staff. Educational financial assistance for formal classes, seminars and conventions help staff members comply with continuing education requirements. These are all good selling points when interviewing job applicants.

It is important that the director of the service and the supervisors make an attempt to provide appropriate management training and impart management philosophy to every staff member. The success of the service depends on the willingness and ability of individual staff members to market the service to patients, to other professionals, and to the community. The staff which understands the goals of the program, the manner in which it contributes to the overall success of the hospital, and the importance of the service to patient care is an invaluable resource for program development.

Establishing a Charge Structure

Determining a charge structure is not an easy task. It is especially difficult for speech-language pathologists and audiologists who are unaccustomed to putting a price on their services. Low-charge structures ultimately affect the quality of services. They also directly affect the salaries paid to speech-language pathologists and audiologists which, in the long run, affect the quality of students who are attracted to our profession. We continue to apologize for charges and we make financial arrangements for payment of our services. It is interesting that families plan to pay privately for orthodontia, dancing lessons and new cars. If a communication problem exists and there is no third-party payor, however, a free clinic is often sought out. Hopefully, future speech-language pathologists and audiologists will be trained to develop appropriate charges, to estimate the duration of the treatment program, and to determine the cost to the patient. Families can then plan for this very important aspect of rehabilitation and feel that it is something worthwhile. This will not occur until the professionals in our fields change their attitudes.

Charges for Speech and Hearing Services

In most departments, charges for speech-language services are based on the amount of time spent with the patient, regardless of the type of patient or the type of communication disorder. The smallest unit of time is usually 30 minutes. The 30-minute charge should be more than half of the 30–60-minute charge. The rationale for this is that the planning and time required to go to the nursing unit and read the chart are the same for a 30-minute session as for a 60-minute session. Many speech-language services find it advantageous to schedule 45-minute sessions. This is an optimal amount of time for many outpatients. Some services have a set charge for evaluations while others base the charge on the time spent. In either case, it is important to consider the time utilized for scoring, interpretation, and reporting. There may be different charges for the treatment of difficult disorders. A uniform treatment charge seems to be more appropriate since the expense involved in providing the treatment is the same regardless of the disorder.

Group versus individual treatments should be considered in the charge structure. The use of group treatment appears to be diminishing due to the emphasis on improved quality of care and the difficulty in finding patients at the same stage of treatment who work well together. Nonetheless, some group treatment continues.

The ideal would be to arrange as much individul treatment as possible with occasional meetings in a small group. Sometimes individual treatment is provided on a regular basis with an additional session of supervised, more independent treatment where on speech-language pathologist assists three or four patients working independently on different assignments. Regardless of the philosophy of grouping patients, it is important that charges are adjusted when more than one patient is seen.

The treatment hour is not an appropriate basis for establishing charges in audiology. Several variables must be taken into account, including staff time per procedure, test interpretation, equipment, maintenance of equipment, space, and supplies. Support personnel may be necessary for patient transport and preparation for highly specialized testing. The counseling time involved in hearing aid fitting and service must be included. A per-procedure charge must be developed that takes these facts into account.

Charges for services provided by graduate interns during a practicum experience must be carefully considered. Each internship is set up differently depending upon the facility. It is recommended that a charge is made only if a staff member is with the intern during a major portion of a treatment session.

Although there are insurance clerks and other business office personnel to assist the patient, the primary responsibility for reimbursement counseling for speech-language pathology and audiology services lies with the professionals involved. The need to stay updated on all types of reimbursement and to know where financial assistance can be obtained for patients cannot be overemphasized. The Health Insurance Manual published by the American Speech-Language-Hearing Association (ASHA) is an excellent resource (1984).

PERSONNEL

All patients with communication disorders must receive evaluation and treatment from a professional holding the Certificate of Clinical Competence (CCC) who assumes responsibility for the management of the problem. Personnel in their clinical fellowship year need special assistance as described in the section on staff supervision. Any other personnel involved with the department must be properly credentialed in their profession. A certified and experienced speech-language pathologist and audiologist should be on the premises when the department is open.

Selection of New Personnel

After working approximately two years in a hospital setting, the speech-language pathologist and audiologist becomes a truly effective and maximally productive staff member. New patients enter into the treatment program almost daily. This fluctuation in patient population and in the work schedule requires flexibility and adaptability on the part of every staff member. From a management standpoint, careful control of patient flow and staffing assignments is directly related to the patient care plan, discharge plan, patient follow-up, and reimbursement.

New graduates beginning the clinical fellowship year in speech-language pathology may be suitable for employment if they have had: (a) appropriate courses in communication disorders related to medical conditions; and (b) an intensive practicum experience in a medical setting. In addition to a proficiency in all routine audiometric tests, successful applicants for an audiology clinical fellowship year position should have experience in hearing aid evaluation and fitting. Experience in test administration and interpretation of both electronystagmography (ENG) and brainstem evoked response (BSER) audiometry is often required.

Certified persons with prior experience in other than hospital settings will require considerable supervision and on-the-job training. Because of the differences that exist among hospitals in the manner in which speech-language pathology and audiology services are organized, managed and delivered, even an experienced hospital person may need an extended period of adjustment when moving to a new position.

Contrasted with professionals in other work settings, speech-language pathologists and audiologists working in hospitals tend to find the intensity level of their job is high. In hospital services that provide outreach consultancies, the staff will have increased responsibility and accountability. Outreach services require extra energy, organization and commitment. Most professionals are willing to accept the additional responsibility because of their interest in providing quality care and developing management skills.

Academic Training

The hospital setting requires basic competencies in all communication disorders associated with specific disease entities, vocal pathologies, congenital anomalies and head trauma. It is important to review a speech-language applicant's transcript in this light. Some specialized information and techniques can be taught on the job if there is a strong academic background. Unfortunately, these types of courses are not required by ASHA. Under present ASHA standards, it is possible for a patient with oral, laryngeal, or pharyngeal cancer to be seen by a certified speech-language pathologist who, in fact, has no academic training nor clinical experience with these disorders.

Other specialized information and skills that are helpful in the hospital setting include: (a) basic information concerning the cardiovascular system and cardiovascular pathologies that affect communication; (b) knowledge of memory processes, perceptual systems, and cognitive processes and their associated communication disorders; (c) basic neurology and central nervous system organization and function; (d) knowledge of geriatrics and common diseases associated with aging; (3) common medications and their effects on behavior; (f) health insurance information; (g) quality assurance mechanisms; (h) knowledge of appropriate medical emergency procedures; (i) familiarity with the roles of various medical and rehabilitation specialties and the ability to relate competently and confidently to them; and (j) evaluating and treating the acutely ill and/or terminally ill patient.

The academic courses required in an ASHA accredited audiology program usually provide a basic level of competence sufficient for work in a hospital. It is important that as much experience as possible is obtained with ENG and BSER at the university or in a practicum at an external site. Additional courses that are helpful include (a) aphasia (b) neurology, (c) organic brain dysfunction, and (d) any courses that will prepare the audiologist for testing the developmentally disabled and psychiatric patient populations.

Desirable Characteristics

It is difficult to determine which speech-language pathologist or audiologist candidate will adapt well to the hospital setting. Experience suggests that certain traists make it easier to work comfortably and effectively. Included in these are (a) flexibility to deal with the constant daily changes which affect most aspects of care; (b) the ability to work independently; (c) willingness to continue to learn; (d) ability to communicate well with families and other professionals who are involved; and (e) readiness to provide coverage and to accept the assignment of a patient not previously seen.

The patient schedule reflects management of time. The entire staff must utilize time effectively, which means stopping and starting according to the designated schedule.

There is no room in the hospital setting for a staff member who needs to be told when to begin work. Speech-language pathologists and audiologists must be ready to initiate programs and be confident and assertive enough to request support services and resources.

Professional credibility is important to the success of the treatment program as well as the overall success of the hospital. All staff members are expected to present a professional appearance in dress and demeanor and to conduct themselves in a professional manner. This includes displaying professional competency, maintaining confidentiality, refraining from gossip and condemnation of the institution and its administration, and any other activities that tend to undermine the morale and the spirit in which services are provided.

It is important to have a position attitude and to attend to any health matter in a timely fashion. The staff member who misses work frequently for health reasons places an additional burden on other staff members who must cover the patient load.

Good writing skills are required because of the number of professional persons providing written documentation on a given patient. Each professional must be able to convey the maximum amount of information in the fewest number of words.

Office Personnel

Secretaries and clerical staff are needed to support the professional workload and are exceedingly important to the success of the services. The skilled secretary-receptionist allows professionals to spend time doing what they are trained to do—the evaluation and treatment of patients. He or she is responsible for scheduling, recording charges for services, obtaining supplies and materials, and compiling many of the monthly statistics and other special reports.

Supportive Personnel

On occasion, the speech-language pathologist and audiologist will be asked to provide training and direction for supportive personnel. Provisions for supportive personnel may be written into government regulations with little or no consultation with the speech-language pathology and audiology profession. Consequently, the positions are poorly defined and have no clearly stated methods for supervision. Nonetheless, these personnel must be used. The director is responsible for clarifying the rules pertaining to supportive personnel and for developing a program that makes effective use of the staff member's time. These factors are important:

1. There is less management control over supportive personnel who are employed by a facility served by the hospital on a contractual basis.
2. A training program must be devised that considers (a) the competency level to be achieved; (b) the length of the training period; (c) whether training is to be provided at the hospital on a short-term intensive basis or provided on the job in the employee's facility; and (d) whether the costs of the training program are included in consultancy charges.
3. The forms to be used by supportive personnel will need to be developed.
4. The extent and nature of documentation to be completed by supportive personnel must be defined.
5. The need for a continuous or ongoing training program should be anticipated because of employee turnover.
6. The ASHA guidelines for supportive personnel will provide direction (ASHA, PSB Manual, 1980).

Graduate Interns

The benefits of an internship in a well-established hospital program cannot be overemphasized. The experience should be viewed as a period of growth in several areas, including (a) the ability to conduct evaluations and to plan treatments for adult patients; (b) the ability to identify a communication problem, break it down into workable components, and formulate specific treatment procedures for each component; (c) the ability to recognize the need to change treatment procedures and techniques; (d) the ability to relate to families of patients with communication disorders; (e) the ability to make decisions, such as formulating prognostic statements, determining the length of treatment and making the decision to terminate treatment; and (f) the opportunity to work alongside several experienced professionals on a daily basis.

Students who have completed all of the required clinical practicum hours before coming to the hospital are free to be involved in a wide variety of those activities that contribute most to furthering their knowledge and broadening their experiences.

The responsibilities and roles of the intern should be defined in a contractual agreement with the training program. This includes a job description and appropriate policies and procedures. The students wear a hospital badge that identifies them as interns. The department staff should be prepared to supervise and share their experiences with the interns.

PROFESSIONAL RELATIONSHIPS

Medical Staff

Credibility is established by providing effective patient services. Channels of communication must be developed so that physicians are aware of what speech-language pathologists and audiologists can do and how well they do it.

Since communication is the essence of professional relationships, it is vital to search continually for ways to improve it, such as: (a) responding promptly to referrals; (b) ensuring that all reports are well-written and promptly completed; (c) offering to telephone results of evaluations to the referring physician prior to sending written reports; (d) providing typed interim treatment summaries that clearly describe patient progress and new treatment objectives; and (e) not suggesting additional medical or hospital services to a patient without first discussing it with the referring physician.

Medical Specialists

Since it is necessary to have the cooperation of the medical staff, it is important to understand the roles of medical specialists. The specialist is a physician who limits practice to a particular area of medicine. At one time most physicians were general practitioners and they provided care for the entire family. With the advancement of medicine in the 1940s, specialization occurred. The speech-language pathologist and audiologist needs to know these specialists:

Specialist in family practice. The general practitioner has been replaced by a residency-trained family physician who is a specialist certified by the American Board of Family Practice. This physician practices internal medicine, pediatrics, obstetrics, psychiatry and public health. Some specialists in family practice do surgery.

Internist. This specialist in Internal Medicine deals with diseases of the internal organs and illness over all of the body.

Otolaryngologist (ENT).   The otolaryngologist treats diseases of the ear, nose and throat.

Neurologist.   The neurologist usually has a specialty in internal medicine and then takes a subspecialty in neurology which deals with functions and disorders of the nervous system.

Neurosurgeon.   The neurosurgeon has a general surgery background and then takes a subspecialty to deal surgically with disorders of the nervous system.

Pediatrician.   This specialist deals with illnesses of the young and growing person.

Orthopedic surgeon.   This is a physician/surgeon who specializes in the prevention, diagnosis and treatment of diseases and abnormalities of the musculoskeletal system.

Physiatrist.   The physiatrist provides and directs the treatment and rehabilitation of the disabled.

Psychiatrist.   The psychiatrist specializes in diagnosis and treatment of disorders of the mind. This physician is involved in the study of emotional processes, their origins and the mental mechanisms underlying them.

Radiologist.   This physician is a specialist in the use of medical science with X-ray (radioactive substances) for the diagnosis and treatment of disease.

In addition to the medical specialties, it is important to understand the contribution of nursing and the other services providing patient care.

Nursing Services

The largest department in the hospital is the nursing service. It is administered by a director of Nursing who may have several associates or assistants.

Regardless of the type of nursing care delivery system, the registered nurse (RN) in charge on each unit is called the head nurse or primary nurse. She may have assistants with varying amounts of training. The RN is accountable for all patients on the unit. The licensed practical nurse (LPN) is under the supervision of the RN and can deliver supportive nursing care. The nurses' aide assists the nurse in activities such as bathing patients and taking pulse and temperature.

Nursing is often the starting point for rehabilitation services. The patient's overall medical care and current status have direct bearing on the treatment procedures speech-language pathology and audiology provide. Nursing continuously assesses the patient's physical condition and provides medical care prescribed by the physician. Nurses who understand the value of speech-language pathology and audiology are more likely to suggest that the physician refer for evaluation and/or treatment. The nursing staff can enhance speech through oral care and by carrying out recommended procedures to facilitate the patient's communication. If the speech-language pathologists provide evaluation and treatment of swallowing disorders, the nurse is an integral part of the dysphagia team. The nursing staff often supplements the basic techniques the patients have learned in the rehabilitation services.

Physical Therapy

The registered physical therapist (RPT) evaluates and assesses a wide variety of disease conditions, musculoskeletal injuries, and pain. Physical conditions treated by the therapist include cardiac and pulmonary care, oncology, pediatrics, wound and burn care, neurological and disease processes, back care, industrial medicine, and athletic injuries. Rehabilitation is achieved through exercise programs to improve strength, movement and coordination. In addition to exercise, pain relief is provided through patient education, mobilization, and physical agents such as heat, cold and electrical stimulation. Physical therapy is an essential part of the rehabilitation process. Speech-language pathology works closely with physical therapy when planning for stroke patients as well as children and adults with neurological disorders. The suggestions of physical therapists provide insight into optimal positioning for respiration and phonation for severe dysarthric patient. They can suggest comfortable sitting or resting positions to increase tolerance for treatment sessions. Information can be shared between disciplines regarding spatial disorientation and body part awareness or neglect. The physical therapist benefits from specific information regarding the patient's communication status, especially the ability to comprehend and follow verbal directions.

Occupational Therapy

The registered occupational therapist (OTR) treats patients who have developmental deficits and disabilities due to aging, physical injury or illness. The OTR helps the patient develop adaptive skills for activities of daily living. The occupational therapist (a) evaluates the patient's potential for self-care skills such as dressing, bathing and feeding; (b) helps with muscle strengthening and coordination of the arms and hands, and provides splinting for weakened arms and hands; (c) assesses the patient's home to reduce barriers and to make the home more adaptive to the patient's abilities; (d) provides help with homemaking skills such as meal preparation, house cleaning and laundry; and (e) orders adaptive devices designed to increase the patient's independence (Special Task Force, 1972).

Speech-language pathologists and occupational therapists work together in developing feeding programs for the dysphagic patient. When videofluoroscopy is used the speech-language pathologist is usually responsible for evaluation and treatment of chewing and swallowing disorders. The occupational therapist may use adaptive devices to help the patient learn to self-feed.

Patients benefit when occupational therapists and speech-language pathologists provide information regarding writing abilities. If the patient does not have a written language disturbance but must learn to write with the nonpreferred hand, the occupational therapist routinely initiates the writing activities. If a written language disturbance is present, the occupational therapist provides the speech-language pathologist with recommendations for body, arm and hand positioning. They also exchange information regarding perceptual problems and their impact on the patient's activities.

Medical Social Work

The medical social worker provides a variety of services for patients in the hospital and/or community. These services generally are divided into four categories: inpatient, outpatient, consultation, and community education services.

Medical social workers provide discharge planning services in consultation with other patient care services and the patient's primary physician.

The social worker has community resource information, including eligibility requirements, service areas, and the populations designated for these resources. Outpatient service programs typically include educational and emotional support groups.

Dietary Services

This department is responsible for the nutritional needs of the hospitalized patient. In addition it provides nutrition education classes and nutrition consultation for various community groups.

The registered dietitian (RD) evaluates and assesses the nutritional status of all patients admitted to the hospital. The dietitian works in conjunction with the physician and other members of the health team to develop a care plan that meets the nutritional goals for the patient.

Hospitalized patients are routinely visited by the dietitians to determine food preferences, tolerance of the diet and the need for diet instruction. Registered dietitians and speech-language pathologists work together to provide evaluation and treatment for patients with disorders of swallowing.

Dietary plays an important role in rehabilitation. The goal is to provide adequate nutritional support to maintain the patient's nutritional status. Recommendations may be made regarding changes for improvement of intake such as consistency of foods, nutritional supplements and ways to stimulate appetite.

Psychology

Psychology services provides testing and psychotherapy for patients and their families. Severe illness or injury often cause disruption of family life and organization, and may result in some significant changes in the attitudes and the behavior of all family members. The psychologist helps the patient adjust to a new lifestyle and assists in setting new vocational and life goals.

Respiratory Care

The respiratory care department provides treatment of patients with pulmonary disease and certain cardiac conditions. These professionals are very helpful in understanding tracheotomies and ventilated patients.

The activities of many additional hospital departments involve the speech-language pathologist and audiologist directly or indirectly.

Medical Records

This department is responsible for release of patient medical information, medical transcription, admission and discharge analyses, and storage and retrieval of records. It assists the hospital and medical staff in record completion and accuracy and it provides advisory services to all professionals regarding record maintenance. Since the prospective payment system (PPS) was implemented, clinical data and financial data are merged for the first time. Medical Records is responsible for coding and assigning diagnosis related categories (DRG) used in the PPS.

Switchboard

The switchboard operator has to know the department's identification and its location. It is poor public relations to have a telephone call come into the switchboard with a request for speech-language pathology or audiology only to be given medical pathology or be told there is no service at that hospital.

Materials Management

This department procures, receives, inventories and distributes all supplies used throughout the hospital. In addition, the department conducts ongoing studies of materials utilization.

Environmental Services (Housekeeping)

Housekeeping maintains the hospital in a sanitary, orderly and attractive condition that meets standards established by the Department of Public Health. It is important to see that they have access to evaluation and treatment areas so their work is not interrupted. If major cleaning is done on weekends and daily cleaning over the noon hour, patient services are not disrupted.

Plant Operations

This department maintains the building, equipment and grounds and ensures safe and efficient operations.

Fiscal Services

In many facilities admitting, accounting, outpatient registration and all billing services are the responsibility of the director of Fiscal Services. This includes everything from patient admission and outpatient registration to the final collection of accounts. Speech-language pathology and audiology have a reasonably complex billing. Problems in any of these areas can mean no reimbursement, dissatisfied "customers," and cancelled consultancies.

MARKETING

Marketing speech-language pathology and audiology services meets a twofold objective: (a) it lets the public and other professionals know that professional services are available in a medical setting; and (b) it increases referrals thereby assuring a sound revenue base for the department. Both are essential to providing the highest quality of care. Quality of care is the most effective marketing tool available.

Market Share

Every geographic area, especially rural areas, has a finite number of people who are potential customers for any service. The same is true for health care services. It is important to know what portion of this group of people can be expected to use the hospital speech-language and hearing services. Several factors determine market share: (a) prevalence of speech-language and hearing problems in the population; (b) geographic area served by the hospital; (c) other sources of speech-language pathology and hearing services in the immediate area; (d) travel distance and time from the farthest points of the market share area to the hospital and the availability of public transportation; (e) age distribution of the population; and (f) available services in contiguous market areas.

Public awareness is essential. A variety of methods and activities that call attention to speech-language and hearing services in the hospital must be developed.

Advertising per se is no longer a controversial issue in health care. It is regarded as a necessary service to the public and a basic component of the professional management of a service. Advertising need not alter the ethical practice of speech-language and hearing services when it is conducted in a professional manner. Yellow page advertising, announcements in the local paper and direct mail should be considered. The best form of advertisement is "word-of-mouth recommendations by a former patient or referral source. It is wise to develop a method of tracking referral sources for new patients. Simply asking them how they happened to come to the department is straight-forward and easy to record.

Marketing Consultancies

The most successful hospital consultancy services are those that operate from a sound departmental base with an established reputation. The success of consultancies depends on (a) a well-trained, experienced staff; (b) thorough knowledge of the rules and regulations affecting the potential consultancy site; (c) available resources to meet the needs of the consultancy; (d) support of the hospital administration for the value of outreach services; (e) support and confidence of the administration of the facility to whom services are provided; and (f) a sound business basis for the consultancy that benefits both the facility, the department and the hospital. Potential targets include nursing homes, small hospitals, sheltered workshops, and facilities for the developmentally disabled.

A successful outreach service benefits all other hospital rehabilitation departments by generating referrals and consultancies for them. Further, it enhances the reputation of the hospital generally and contributes to the institutional marketing effort.

CONCLUSION

The phenomenal growth of hospital-based services clearly characterizes the maturation of our profession, and that process is continuing. Entering the health care field has and will continue to force changes in our attitudes and our practices. The wisdom and foresight of our professional association have given us the opportunities for a strong and viable professional position in health care. That position is established and maintained by the day-to-day management performed by each of us who chooses to work in these settings. Dr. Jerry Griffith has summed up our task in these words:

> There is not a single work setting for speech-language pathologists or audiologists where you can assume that someone else will look after your affairs. In your professional life, as in your personal life, you are the product of your own self-management skills (Personal communication, Sept., 1983).

There is no other setting in which this is more true than in health care.

REFERENCES

AMERICAN HOSPITAL ASSOCIATION (1985). *AMH/86 accreditation manual for hospitals.* Chicago, Ill.

AMERICAN HOSPITAL ASSOCIATION. (1985). *Hospital statistics.* Chicago, Ill.

AMERICAN MEDICAL ASSOCIATION. (1978). *Allied health education directory* (7th ed.). Chicago, Ill.

AMERICAN SPEECH-LANGUAGE-HEARING ASSOCIATION. (1984). *Manual of professional services board (PSB).* Rockville, Md.

BALICK, S., G. GREEN, J. KAPLAN, D. PRESS, AND J. DEMOPOULOS. (1978). "The problem-oriented medical record applied to communicative disorders," *Archives of Physical Medicine and Rehabilitation, 59,* 288–289.

BECK, D. (1980). *Basic hospital financial management.* Rockville, Md.: Aspen.

BOUCHARD, M. AND H. SHANE. (1977). "Use of the problem-oriented medical record in the speech and hearing profession," *Asha, 19* (3), 157–159.

DOUNEY, M. S. WHITE AND S. KARR. (1984). *Health insurance manual.* Rockville, Md.: American Speech-Language-Hearing Association.

DRUCKER, P. (1974). *Management: Tasks, responsibilities, practices.* New York: Harper and Row.

GRIFFITH, J. AND T. STRANDBERG. (1982). *A guide to nursing home living.* Charleston, Ill.: Generations Publishing.

HAIMANN, T. (1973). *Supervisory management for health care*. St. Louis, MO.: Catholic Hospital Association.

LOAVENBRUCK, A. AND J. MADELL. (1981). *Hearing and dispensing for audiologists*. New York: Grune and Stratton, 1981.

ROWLAND, H. AND B. ROWLAND. *Hospital management: A guide to departments*. Rockville, Md.: Aspen.

SARAH BUSH LINCOLN HEALTH CENTER. (1983). *Procedures manual for budget process*. Mattoon, Ill.

SPECIAL TASK FORCE. (1972). "Occupational therapy: Its definition and functions," *American Journal of Occupational Therapy, 26* (4), 204–205.

STRANDBERG, T. (1977). "A national study of United States hospital speech pathology services, report number one," *Asha, 19* (2), 69–76.

STRANDBERG, T. (1977). "A national study of United States hospital speech pathology services, report number two," *Asha, 19* (3), 160–163.

WHITE, STEVEN C. (1986). "Joint commission for the accreditation of hospitals—1986 rehabilitation standards." *Asha, 28* (4), 25–27.

8 Administration of a Military-Based Program of Speech-Language Pathology and Audiology

Roy K. Sedge*

INTRODUCTION

Provision of speech-language and hearing services in the military community provides a unique model of socialized health care. Unlike the diverse, decentralized models seen in the civilian community, military medical services are centrally administered. Military health care administration is guided by a series of standardized regulations directed by congressional policy. Policy matters affecting health services are referred to the respective armed forces surgeons general for implementation. It is at this point in the military system that actual management of speech-language and hearing services begin.

Programs for speech-language and hearing services currently exist in all branches of the tri-services, i.e., army, navy and air forces. Although differing in size and scope all are centrally administered. To maintain accuracy concerning pertinent regulations and to avoid confusion concerning delivery models among the tri-services, it should be noted that this chapter is written from an army perspective.

*Ltc. Sedge, Ph.D., is director, Army Audiology and Speech Center, Walter Reed Army Medical Center, and consultant in Audiology to the chief of the Medical Service Corps and to the Army Surgeon General. (The opinions or assertions contained herein are the private view of the author and are not to be construed as official or as reflecting the views of the Department of the Army or the Department of Defense.)

In general, however, the navy and air forces programs are parallel in several administrative areas.

The administrative procedures for speech-language and hearing programs described in this chapter are based on numerous army regulations. While the chapter provides a generalized overview of the administration of these programs, specific guidelines for the army's policies are clearly outlined in the regulations. The interested reader is referred to appendix I for a listing of pertinent army regulations.

Historical Overview

Management practices for speech-language and hearing services in the military and in the private sector have evolved from early pioneer work in rehabilitation programs for deaf and hard-of-hearing service members. In fact, rehabilitation services for deaf service members preceded the commercial development of the hearing aid. In World War I, a lipreading school was established at Hospital Number 11 in Cape May, New Jersey, staffed by "eleven experts in the field" (Morrisett, 1957). Soldiers who could not hear conversational speech at a distance of five feet were instructed in the art of lipreading. Instruction was individualized except for group practice work. Classes, which were held in private rooms without distraction, met two or three times daily for sessions of 30–45 minutes each. Teachers rotated among classes so patients would gain experience in reading a variety of lip shapes and conversational patterns. Instruction continued until the soldier "reached a level of ability as a lipreader beyond which further improvement did not seem likely." A total of 108 war-deafened soldiers received instruction during the school's year of operation. Due to the reported lack of methods for identifying hearing loss an estimated 400 additional untreated soldiers were returned to civilian life.

During World War II, an army medical manual described the original lip reading program as "one of the bright spots in the army's reconstruction activities." Dr. Gordon Berry (1942) summed up the World War I program by stating: "The remarkably short time required to acquire the art of lipreading is ascribed to three factors: (1) the intensive nature of the work, (2) the individual lessons, and (3) the enthusiasm and persuasiveness of the highly skilled teachers. The men were saturated with lipreading in an optimistic environment of devoted service. The nearer one can approach such an intensive program in such an environment, the better will be the results" (p. 257). This premise set the stage for development of the present army aural rehabilitation system since casualties from World War II brought renewed interest in hearing and speech rehabilitation. On 28 May, 1943 the army designated specialized centers for the treatment of service members having "defective hearing of a degree which precluded the return of the patient to duty." These centers were established at Borden General Hospital, Chickasha, Oklahoma; Hoff General Hospital, Santa Barbara, California; and Walter Reed General Hospital, Washington, D.C. Because of the inpatient caseload at Walter Reed, rehabilitation duties were transferred to Deshon General Hospital, Butler, Pennsylvania. To oversee the operation of the aural rehabilitation programs, an otolaryngologic branch was established in the army surgeon general's office in July of 1944. In Canfield's (1957) account of the administrative aspects of otolaryngology in World War II it is stated that "the impetus for creation of the branch at this time was the reorganization of the Aural Rehabilitation Program for the deafened and hard of hearing" (p. 383). Canfield further states that until the end of World War II, the activities of the consultant in otolaryngology were directed almost entirely to that program: "His responsibilities for otolaryngology in general being incidental to his duties in connection with the Aural Rehabilitation Program."

A conference on rehabilitation of the hard-of-hearing soldier was held at Hoff General Hospital in February 1944. The proceedings of the conference founded the modern principles of aural rehabilitation. The conference included otolaryngologists, principals of the aural rehabilitation programs, staff, hearing aid experts and invited guests. All phases of rehabilitation were addressed, including medical-nonmedical treatment, administration, equipment, course content and fitting rationales for hearing aids. The results of the conference were put into recommendations and eventually became the basic policy for administration of audiology and speech-language and hearing services in the military today. The most relevant recommendations were that:

1. Rehabilitation services for the deaf (and hard-of-hearing) be independent of otolaryngologic sections.
2. Trained personnel be left undisturbed in the rehabilitation services.
3. Otologists, lipreading teachers and other personnel be supplied in proportion to patient loads.
4. Hearing aids be furnished to all deafened and hard-of-hearing in the army instead of, as at present, only to men with hearing impairment incurred in the line of duty.
5. Training in residual hearing, psychiatric examinations and vocational rehabilitation be stressed.
6. Certain administrative changes be made including the appointment of a superintendent of the rehabilitative services at each center, to coordinate the work of the program and to direct all administrative and nonmedical activities.

Lack of standardized clinical test procedures also created difficulty. For example, nonuniform test protocols for determination of patients' hearing sensitivity created confusion in diagnosis and treatment. Dr. Walter Hughson deplored the lack of standardization and called for objective tests by qualified personnel to determine status, potential and progress of patients with hearing disorders (Morrisett, 1957). Dr. Hughson's efforts in standardizing rehabilitation programs were realized in late 1944 when the surgeon general recommended that all centers be organized in a similar manner. Figure 8-1 illustrates their common structure. This organizational structure can be seen in today's larger military programs. Titles, however, have changed. Acoustic physicists, lipreading instructors, aural rehabilitation officers and speech correction instructors are the audiologists and speech-language pathologists of today. In 1946 the army's rehabilitation officers' activities were consolidated at

GENERAL PLAN OF ORGANIZATION
FOR WORLD WAR II ARMY AURAL
REHABILITATION CENTERS

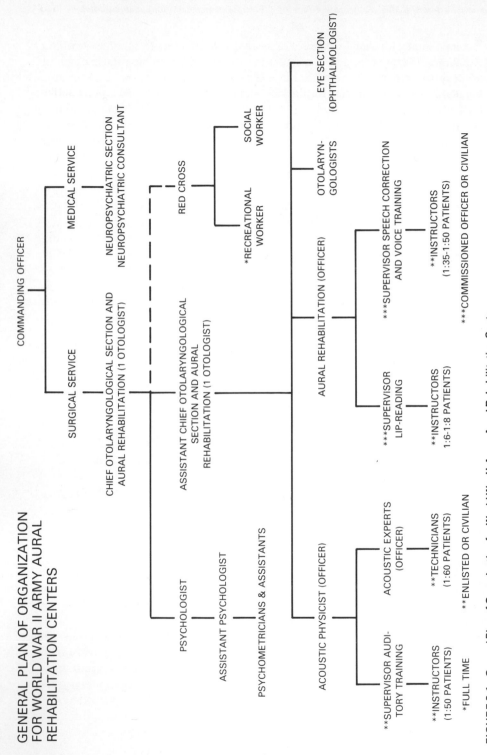

FIGURE 8-1 General Plan of Organization for World War II Army Aural Rehabilitation Centers.
(Morrissett, 1957)

the Army Audiology and Speech Center, Walter Reed General Hospital, now Walter Reed Army Medical Center. To this day, this center remains the principal site of audiology and speech rehabilitation activities within the army.

Rehabilitation activities for the following twenty years focused around activities at Walter Reed and at other army medical centers with otolaryngology resident training programs. Audiology and speech-language pathology staff consisted of civilians hired by each individual facility. Although there were a few audiologists who served on active duty prior to 1965, they were actually assigned to other career specialties. Because of the diverse military needs for military audiologists, (for example, clinicians, hearing conservationists, rehabilitationists and researchers) pressure was brought to bear on the Army Medical Department to create an occupational specialty for audiology officers.

In January 1966, the military audiology specialty was formally established. Audiology officers were called upon to develop clinical programs at the larger teaching hospitals. Duties included diagnostic audiology, rehabilitative audiology and resident training. At the time that the army audiology officer specialty was created, the Army Medical Department formulated a policy statement which was subsequently printed in *ASHA Magazine* concerning speech-language-pathologists (ASHA editorial staff, 1967). Unfortunately, the statement is still in effect. "The army has no plans to establish a specialty for speech pathologists. Reasons given for this decision are that individuals with serious speech disorders are not taken into the army initially, and if a speech disorder develops during army service it is usually associated with other physical problems which result in discharge from military service and follow-up care through the Veterans Administration or other facilities. Where the army does provide speech pathology services for example at the Army Medical Center or at army hospitals serving dependents, it is felt that this can be done most efficiently through the use of civilian speech pathologists in civil service positions" (p. 11).

By 1967 the army had created eleven positions for audiologists (Northern and Endicott, 1968). The number of audiologists grew slowly. It was apparent that the number of service members suffering noise-induced hearing losses had increased to an unacceptable level. An epidemiological study initiated in 1972 documented that as many as 50 percent of soldiers in the combat arms suffered some measurable hearing loss (Walden, et al., 1975). The army chief of staff determined that this was unacceptable, particularly since prevention was possible. Within two years, the number of audiology officers increased to fifty-eight. As of 1985 approximately seventy officers serve as audiologists in the army.

Roles for military audiologists and their civilian counterparts have changed significantly since 1966. Officers today are expected to divide their time evenly between clinical duties and administration of local hearing conservation programs at their installation. Positions have also been established for both military and civilian audiologists in the areas of research and administration, as well as in other activities in the health care system.

Military Medical Philosophy that Guides Administration

Administration of speech-language and hearing services in the military is guided by a central administrative structure which begins with and is dictated by congressional policy. The major principle that guides all administrative and clinical decisions in the army's health care system is "to conserve the fighting strength." This principle is one of the major factors for having audiologic and speech-language services in the army today. One will recall that early efforts were rehabilitative in nature. Today, prevention is the first concern. The overall preservation of health is a vital element if service members are to work to their capacity. In this context, those eligible for military health care services (active duty, retired military and their dependents) are afforded the most comprehensive health care available. Generally, political doctrine pertaining to the army is conveyed by the secretary of defense to the army chief of staff through the Secretary of the Army. Matters of health care are directed to the army surgeon general, the principal advisor for all health care matters, by the army chief of staff.

The Army Medical Department

Health care for the army community is directed by the army surgeon general who oversees the Army Medical Department (AMEDD). Since a complex system of health care requires an extensive mix of specialty personnel, the AMEDD is separated into six separate corps to provide an orderly grouping of health care functions. These include the Army Medical Corps, the Army Dental Corps, the Army Nurse Corps, the Army Medical Specialist Corps, and the Medical Service Corps. Each is directed by a chief who is administratively and technically responsible to the surgeon general. A specific corps may be composed of one or more broad health professional disciplines. For example, the Medical Service Corps is divided into the following:

a. Pharmacy, Supply and Administration
    1. Aeromedical evacuation
    2. Health services comptrollership
    3. Health care administration
    4. Health services plans and operations
    5. Health services personnel management
    6. Pharmacy
    7. Patient administration
    8. Health care logistics
    9. Biomedical information systems
    10. Health facilities planning
    11. Health services manpower control
    12. Field medicine
b. Medical Allied Sciences
    1. Audiology
    2. Laboratory sciences
    3. Podiatry

      4. Psychology
      5. Social work
   c. Sanitary Engineering
      1. Sanitary engineering
      2. Environmental science
      3. Entomology
      4. Nuclear medical science
   d. Optometry

Audiology officers are part of the Medical Allied Sciences Section of Medical Service Corps. The corps consists of the chief who is a brigadier general, and four assistant chiefs heading the Pharmacy, Supply and Administration Section, the Allied Sciences Section, the Sanitary Engineering Section and the Optometry Section. Each section is composed of a broad series of health care disciplines. Officers in the Medical Service Corps, including audiologists, are normally utilized in their broad area of professional training. They may also, if qualified, provide administrative support to clinical care operations, actively engage in research and provide professional support in health and environmental activities.

THE HEALTH SERVICE COMMAND AND OTHER HEALTH CARE ACTIVITIES

Audiology officers may be assigned to a variety of military installations within different army medical commands. The structure of the army's commands and the health care services within these commands frequently dictate the number of audiologists assigned to a given installation/activity as well as the job responsibilities they have.

Health Service Command

The Health Service Command (HSC) is a major army command which provides administrative supervision and control for all fixed medical facilities in the United States. The Office of the Surgeon General generates policy and manages personnel within the Army Medical Department. The Health Service Command, on the other hand, administrates the health care facilities in accordance with stated policy.

To provide overall continuity of health care in the United States, Health Service Command has divided the country into seven health service regions (HSR), (fig. 8–2a). The organization of each health service region is similar (fig. 8–2b). Health Service Command directives originate from the Health Service Command commander (commands are commanded by commanders) who has intermediate advisors who are commanders of the seven medical centers (MEDCEN). These commanders are coordinators for health care activities within their health service region. A staff of specialty consultants, generally chiefs of their services within the MEDCEN,

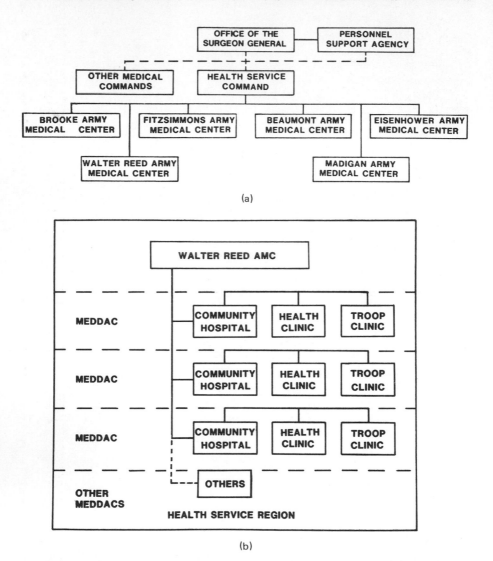

FIGURE 8-2 Command Structure, Health Services Command, and Health Service Region.

serve each commander and provide staff visits and consultation services for appropriate facilities within the region. Coordination is also provided for continuing education and quality assurance assistance. Specialty consultants such as audiologists are expected to visit each hospital within the region on an annual basis.

Each health service region is subdivided into medical activities (MEDDAC). The community hospital is the focal point within each MEDDAC providing specialty support and consultation services to outlying community health and troop clinics.

The community hospital specialty health care professional discusses MEDDAC activities with the MEDCEN specialty consultant. On an annual basis, the MEDCEN specialty consultant summarizes all MEDDAC activities within the health service region and forwards a report through the regional coordinator to Health Service Command for evaluation. Annual reports reflect the need for changes in services provided, addition or reduction of personnel as a result of mission changes, need for additional space and equipment, and a review of quality assurance measures. Perhaps the most practical advantage of continuous specialty support is that contact is maintained between more isolated health care personnel and their professional colleagues. An audiology specialty consultant is available within each health service region to advise the regional commander and provide support to audiologists assigned within the region. The commander of Health Service Command in turn has an audiology consultant to provide assistance on overall matters.

THE STRUCTURE OF AUDIOLOGY AND SPEECH LANGUAGE SERVICES WITHIN THE COMMAND

Audiologic care exists at three levels and speech-language services at two levels within each health service region. The most basic of audiologic services are conducted at auditory screening clinics. Pure tone air conduction threshold examinations are provided at these clinics to patients receiving care for minor illness and in support of the post hearing conservation program. Auditory screening clinics are located within troop clinics and army health clinics throughout individual MEDDACs. Troop medical clinics provide limited treatment for service members directly within their work area. Patients with more serious problems are referred to the local community hospital or army health clinic. Unlike the troop medical clinic the health clinic is designed, equipped and staffed to provide ambulatory health care services. On occasion the auditory screening clinic located within the health clinic will provide a basic audiologic battery to include air and bone conduction, speech and immittance measures.

The second level of audiologic and first level of speech-language care is provided at an auditory diagnostic clinic (ADC). A wide range of diagnostic audiologic and speech-language services are available. ADCs are located in a United States community hospital. In addition, these facilities generally have the ability to support up to 200 inpatients and to provide definitive outpatient care. The hospital is staffed and equipped to provide diagnostic and therapeutic services in the field of general medicine and surgery and to provide extensive preventive medicine services.

The third echelon of audiology and the second echelon of speech-language care in a health service region are provided at an auditory evaluation and treatment clinic (AETC), located at army medical centers (MEDCEN). These clinics provide the most extensive range of hearing and speech services in the region. AETCs provide hearing aid and aural rehabilitation services. It will be recalled that auditory diagnostic clinics do not provide hearing aids and aural rehabilitation services. The rationale for division of diagnostic and rehabilitation between auditory diagnostic clinics and auditory treatment clinics is based on the nature of the population supported. Audiology services at community hospitals, as will be seen in a later section of this chapter, are focused on the prevention of hearing loss. Medical centers and their AETCs are generally located away from troop concentrations and emphasis is on the more time consuming rehabilitative aspects of health care.

Medical centers are large teaching hospitals ranging from 500 to 1,200 beds. They are equipped and staffed to provide a wide range of specialized and consultative support functions for the health service region. The staff administers specialty residency programs provide postgraduate seminars and conduct training programs in allied health professions.

The highest echelon of hearing, speech and language care in the army is provided at the Army Audiology and Speech Center (AASC), Walter Reed Army Medical Center (WRAMC). This center provides care for patients referred from other medical centers and facilities throughout the army and the Department of Defense. Unlike other AETCs, the Army Audiology and Speech Center provides inpatient services for aural rehabilitation and special speech-language problems. The Army Audiology and Speech Center also serves as a coordinating agency for all of the AETCs, features a hearing aid repair section as well as an active applied research program, and provides training to new army audiologists.

Health Care Activities Supported by Audiologists

Audiologists are utilized in managing the overall army hearing conservation program and conducting research on the effects of noise and human performance. The Bioacoustics Division (BAD) of the United States Army Environmental Hygiene Agency (USAEHA) is the principal resource facility for all army hearing conservation activities. Army audiologists in the division conduct individual program evaluations and provide ongoing technical support to hearing conservation audiologists. (A detailed discussion of the Bioacoustics Division's function is contained elsewhere in this chapter.) As a member of a research team, audiologists at the United States Army Aeromedical Research Laboratories (USAARL), which is part of the United States Army Medical Research and Development Command, investigate the effectiveness of hearing protective and communication devices utilized in aircraft and other equipment.

The Human Engineering Laboratories (HEL) is a research and development command located at the United States Army Environmental Hygiene Agency. Multidiscipline research teams investigate the practical problems of equipment operators communicating in typical noise environments. Audiologists are also active in research involving the nonauditory effects of blast overpressure.

MANAGEMENT OF AUDIOLOGY AND SPEECH LANGUAGE SERVICES IN ARMY FACILITIES

Army audiology officers administer hearing conservation and clinical activities in a variety of work settings. The following section describes the administrative aspects of audiology and speech-language pathology programs and hearing conservation programs in medical as well as nonmedical facilities.

Management within Medical Facilities

In keeping with the army's philosophy "to conserve the fighting strength," audiologists are primarily involved with protecting the hearing of active duty service members. Hearing conservation activities, especially the audiologic monitoring aspects, are conducted in auditory screening clinics. While overall control of the auditory screening clinic is the responsibility of the chief of the troop medical clinic or community health clinic, the audiologist in the army community hospital is responsible for providing technical consultation and supervising technicians conducting the audiologic examinations. In addition, they are also responsible for technical aspects of test administration, equipment calibration, and test interpretation for the clinic chief. Accurate audiometric tests are facilitated by the extensive use of microprocessor-controlled audiometers. Software programs, specifically written to match hearing loss with army profiling standards, aid in making appropriate referrals.

When indicated, the patient is referred from the auditory screening clinic for a more extensive audiologic workup at the audiology diagnostic clinic at the local community hospital. These clinics are generally equipped for complete audiologic evaluations including auditory brainstem responses, and electronystagmography. An otolaryngologist is available for referral. When medical treatment is not indicated, patients in need of amplification are referred to the medical center supporting that community hospital for a hearing aid evaluation and aural rehabilitation. Prior to transferring the patient, medical and audiologic workups including earmold impressions are completed. When the patient arrives at the medical center's auditory evaluation and treatment clinic, all records and custom earmolds are available.

Speech-language services in the diagnostic clinics parallel those in the auditory evaluation and treatment clinics. Services are provided for local outpatients and short-term inpatients. Long-term speech pathology cases are referred to the Veterans' Administration Hospital system or to a civilian convalescent facility. Because speech-language services to school age children are provided within the school system these services are not typically provided at the auditory diagnostic clinic.

Audiology diagnostic clinics are usually a division of the Otolaryngology Service. Depending on the population served, the service will minimally include one otolaryngologist, one audiologist, one speech-language pathologist, two technicians, and clerical support. If the population is extremely large additional staff may be necessary. (See "Staffing Requirements," later in this chapter) As a rule of thumb one audiologist is required for every ten thousand active duty troops served. One speech-language pathologist is generally sufficient to support the community hospital. While the audiologist is accountable to and receives indirect supervision from the chief of Otolaryngology, technical supervision is provided by the regional consultant. Supervision becomes especially confusing for audiologists who spend 50 percent of their time in hearing conservation activities which are administered by the Preventive Medicine officer. Which master is served? A unique three-tiered rating system provides a check and balance system in order to rate the performance of the audiologist fairly. Either the chief of Otolaryngology or the chief of Preventive Medicine first rates the audiologist while the other officer acts as an intermediate rater. A third and more senior staff member (for example, chief of Professional Services, Chief of Department of Surgery) verifies the accuracy of the report. Civilian audiologists and speech-language pathologists are supervised by the military audiologist who is the section chief. A factor which further complicates the supervision picture is military rank. In some cases the army audiologist will outrank the otolaryngologist. The chief of surgery will then directly supervise both officers.

One will recall that an auditory evaluation and treatment clinic provides the third echelon of audiology and speech-language pathology care. These clinics provide hearing aid fittings and aural rehabilitation as well as those functions also performed at the first- and second-level echelon clinics. Since a broader range of services is provided, AETCs by necessity have larger staffs. There are eight AETCs in the army medical system. The administrative structure at AETCs is similar to those in the auditory diagnostic clinics.

The Army Audiology and Speech Center is the highest echelon of speech-language-hearing care in the Department of the Army. It functions as an independent service within the Department of Surgery at the Walter Reed Army Medical Center. The director, an army audiologist, is responsible for all personnel actions, budget, clinic policy and space allocations. Administratively, the director reports to the chief of the Department of Surgery and coordinates clinic activities with the chief of Otolaryngology. In addition, the director is the audiology consultant to the surgeon general and the chief of the Medical Service Corps.

Management of the Army Hearing Conservation Program

Military audiologists are on active duty primarily as hearing conservation managers. Two critical elements are necessary for a successful hearing conservation program: (1) a regulation that describes the essential elements of the program, and (2) a manager of the overall operation. The army's program has these critical elements. The regulation governing the program is the Department of Defense Instruction (DoDI 6055.3), Hearing Conservation. The Bioacoustics Division of the Army Environmental Hygiene Agency (AEHA) oversees the program.

In 1978, Department of Defense (DoD) regulations spelling out the elements of hearing conservation programs were promulgated. The Bioacoustics Division also instituted a data management program for the audiometric data of all army personnel working in noise hazardous areas.

Although the DoD regulation was written for tri-services hearing conservation programs, management was left to each individual branch. Audiologists were selected to serve as program managers in each service. Under guidance set forth by the respective surgeons general, all military hearing conservation programs must include the following features: (1) noise measurement analysis; (2) caution signs and warning labels; (3) noise abatement measures; (4) provision for personal hearing protection devices; (5) education; (6) audiometric testing; (7) personnel preselection criteria; and (8) record keeping. Army personnel who manage the hearing conservation programs have been trained as hearing conservation technicians and course directors using the standards developed by the Council on Accreditation of Occupational Hearing Conservation (CAOHC). New personnel who are not certified must attend a hearing conservation certification workshop prior to managing a hearing conservation program. These workshops are administered by CAOHC-accredited army audiology course directors.

Under the army's guidelines, all personnel exposed to 85 dBA of noise in the workplace are automatically entered into the hearing conservation program. Although provisions may exist for time/intensity tradeoffs for other services, the army opted to utilize a fixed intensity level. Supervision of personnel involved in programs utilizing time/intensity tradeoffs was felt to be ineffective. Administratively the programs were not feasible.

Personal hearing protective devices are medically fitted to all service members entering active duty. Audiologists at basic training posts oversee the fitting program. Audiometric data management is an interactive process involving the post audiologist and the Bioacoustics Division. Baseline audiograms are obtained for all service members entering active duty. This document serves as a comparison for all subsequent hearing conservation audiograms throughout the service member's military career. Triplicate copies of the baseline and annual hearing conservation audiograms are made. One copy is sent to the Bioacoustics Division, another is maintained at the local installation and the final copy is placed in the service member's personal health record. Whenever a threshold shift of 20 dB or more occurs in either ear at any test frequency relative to the individual's baseline audiogram, referral is made for medical evaluation and counseling. Should the threshold shift be permanent, the individual may be flagged for administrative action, that is, job reclassification or reassignment. Measures are also taken to determine any source of failure in the program and to institute corrective actions.

The Bioacoustics Division of the Army Environmental Hygiene Agency

Support of the army hearing conservation program is the major function of the Bioacoustics Division. The division's services are available to all army commands and individual installations, and it carries out activities on a worldwide basis. Managed by an army audiologist, the division conducts hearing conservation surveys on a scheduled basis, and runs hearing conservation workshops for technicians and for future course directors. The division maintains a data repository for all noise-hazardous equipment utilized in the army. Physical onsite inspection of each individual hearing conservation program is another task of the division. Continuity between the division and individual hearing conservation program managers is facilitated by training all new audiology officers when they first come on active duty. Once the audiologist is assigned to a particular post, a Bioacoustic Division audiology team visits the program and provides any necessary consultation assistance. After the audiologist has worked in the program for a time, the installation is revisited and formally evaluated by division representatives. The report lists strengths, weaknesses and the corrective actions necessary for the program to be in compliance with army standards.

The Bioacoustics Division is an excellent resource for the hearing conservation audiologist. In addition to its consulting functions the division prepares necessary technical guidelines for hearing conservation and provides education materials necessary to conduct an effective hearing conservation program.

Hearing Evaluation Automated Registry System

Despite intensive management of hearing conservation programs, it is still difficult to measure the efficacy of a program. Ideally, a successful hearing conservation program should safeguard the service members' hearing for as long as they remain on active duty. In other words, in the absence of pathology, hearing sensitivity of service members should remain stable. Presbycusis is not a major factor since the average retirement age is 42.2 years of age. With the vast number of individuals on active duty, and the transient nature of the occupation, management of audiometric data is difficult. The Bioacoustics Division has developed a computerized central repository for hearing conservation audiograms to facilitate control.

The data sent to the agency by all army hearing conservation programs is entered into the Hearing Evaluation Automated Data Registry System (HEARS). In addition to audiometric data, other information is sent, including the service member's occupation, tester identification, and type of hearing protection being used. Thus, at any time in the service member's career any audiogram on the computer can be measured against baseline. Individual and group trends can be objectively measured. The HEARS is a new concept. In the future these data will also provide objective answers to individual noise susceptibility, effectiveness of individual post hearing conservation programs, and a multitude of other data with which to enhance the effectiveness of the army's hearing conservation efforts.

PERSONNEL PROCUREMENT AND DEVELOPMENT

Speech and hearing services in the military are administered by trained professionals. The army employs approximately seventy audiology officers. Additionally, some seventy speech-language pathology positions and a comparable number of audiology positions are available to civilians.

Audiology Officer Procurement

There is a small but steady demand for army audiology officers. Due to retirements, separations and new positions, approximately six to eight new vacancies become available each year. Individuals who accept an army officer's commission are obligated for a three-year tour of duty. An applicant must possess a master's degree from an accredited program that is recognized by the Army Medical Department. Priority is given to applicants graduating from university programs that are accredited by the Educational Standards Board of the American Speech-Language Hearing Association. If an individual receives a commission through ROTC and has completed a master's program in audiology, an assignment as an army audiologist is usually provided. ROTC candidates do not, however, fill all of the audiology positions. In fact, the vast majority of audiologists enter active duty with a direct commission. Applicants entering active duty in this manner are selected by a board of officers. Applications are available at Army Medical Department procurement offices located throughout the United States. (These agencies are not to be confused with the army recruitment centers that primarily seek applicants in enlisted military grades.) Applications include a description of academic experience, past employment experience, letters of recommendation, national security checks, a statement of interest by the applicant, and a physical examination. The army audiology consultant reviews each application and when possible interviews the applicant. A recommendation is made to the selection board based on the aforementioned considerations. A personnel officer also reviews the record to insure its administrative completeness. Applications are forwarded to the board, which typically convenes three times a year. Applications are ranked on a best-qualified basis and a specific number of the top applicants based on the number of vacancies are offered a direct commission.

Civilian Speech-Language-Hearing Procurement

In addition to army audiology officer positions, there is also a steady demand for civilian speech-language pathologists and audiologists in the army. Individuals seeking employment in the army apply in the same manner as all federal applicants in speech-language pathology and audiology. Applications are submitted to the Office of Personnel Management. Special examining units rate the application and place the applicant's name on a federal register. When positions become available, applicants are referred on a best-qualified basis. Individuals appear on the register in the order of their rating. The employer must interview the top applicants first. If none of the applicants is appropriate for the position the employer interviews others from the register until a qualified individual is found. This selection process is designed to identify the best applicant on an impartial basis while permitting each employer to select an individual who best meets the needs of a specific position.

Officer Professional Development

The careers of audiology officers are centrally managed through interactions with the audiology consultant and the Medical Service Corps career activities officer. Audiology officers have the opportunity to chart their professional development.

Through the director of Personnel, the surgeon general manages the procurement, training, assignment, promotion and final separation/retirement phases of each officer's military career. Management is conducted by individual specialty. The Medical Service Corps is responsible for overall management of army audiologists.

As in all careers, the individual is the most critical and responsible element in determining his or her professional career objectives. No matter how skilled the individual becomes as an audiologist, managerial skills are becoming increasingly necessary for career progression. In this respect, the term *dual career* is often used with health care professionals. This means that one's chosen civilian profession is, in effect, intertwined with that of a military profession. For the army audiologist, professional responsibilities are integrated with the army health care system. Officers are expected to pursue continuing education in both the professional and military elements of their career. A structured four-phase career program is followed by each audiology officer through guidance and mediation with the audiology consultants and career activity officers (See Table 8-1). The first phase, called the *basic professional development period*, covers the period from entry onto active duty through the seventh year of service. The audiologist may initially be assigned to a variety of duties which largely depend on prior clinical experience and clinical certification status. In an interactive process, the officer, the audiology consultant, and the career activities officer review career progression options and determine the most appropriate moves for each officer's career development. Often assignments are made with the next assignment in mind. Since each of the first three assignments in an officer's career is generally a three-year tour, careers can be charted in advance. As experience is gained, assignment rotations may occur less often. As assignments become more complex, additional time may be necessary to carry out long-term management objectives. During the basic professional development period, audiologists' training is focused on developing a strong working knowledge of their role in the army's overall health care team. Emphasis is placed on developing administrative skills as an action officer for hearing conservation, as well as clinical skills. Audiologists who have just completed their graduate training programs are generally placed in a position with an experienced audiology supervisor. The junior member can then develop diagnostic and rehabilitation skills as well as managerial skills in hearing conservation, while completing requirements for clinical certification. Those who come on active duty with prior professional experience and certification may be placed in nonsupervised programs. They may supervise a civilian audiologist as well.

During the basic professional development period focus is also placed on fundamental military training. Prior to their first duty assignment all newly appointed officers attend an Army Medical Department basic course at Fort Sam Houston, Texas, headquarters of Health Service Command. After this nine-week orientation course on the fundamental aspects of the army health care structure, they attend an audiology training course at the Army Audiology and Speech Center, and hearing conservation training at the Bioacoustics Division. At their initial post installation the officers are also exposed to military, clinical and managerial practices in support hospital and hearing conservation programs. Officers who wish to

TABLE 8-1 Audiology Officer Career Development Planning Guide

				PROFESSIONAL DEVELOPMENT GUIDE		AUDIOLOGIST	
YEAR	PHASES OF DEVELOPMENT	PROFESSIONAL DEVELOPMENT OBJECTIVES	ASSIGNMENTS	OFFICER PROFESSIONAL EDUCATION			YEAR
				PROFESSIONAL MILITARY EDUCATION	SPECIALTY EDUCATION		
30							30
29	MAJOR PROFESSIONAL CONTRIBUTION PERIOD (Over 23 years)	Maximum utilization through assignments of increasing responsibility as determined by demonstrated ability. Exceptionally qualified officers are awarded 9A ASI			CONTINUING EDUCATION THROUGHOUT CAREER		29
28							28
27							27
26							26
25							25
24					SHORT COURSES		24
23			Chief Audiologist MEDCEN, CHIEF, Audiology Research Team, Audiology Consultant OTSG, MEDCOMEUR, H3C, Chief, Research Audiologist USARMRDC, Director Army Audiology Speech Center	National War College, Army War College, Industrial College of the Armed Forces			23
22							22
21	ADVANCED CONTRIBUTION AND DEVELOPMENT PERIOD (15-23 years)	Provide leasership for audiology programs in key assignments, contribute to advancement of science through research, participation in national organizations, and contributions to literature. Qualified officers are awarded 9B ASI					21
20							20
19							19
18							18
17					CONFERENCES		17
16							16
15			Chief, Audiologist MEDCAN, Audiology Consultant to Command or Agency, Chief, Audiologist USAMRDC.				15
14							14
13		Develop level of professional competence to allow independent action. Develop ability to instruct AMEDD officer and enlisted personnel in principles and practice of audiology / hearing conservation. Develop skill in coordinating audiology activities with other AMEDD elements. Make contribution to advancement of profession. Qualified officers are awarded 9C ASI		Command & General Staff College; Armed Forces Staff College	PROFESSIONAL MEETINGS		13
12	INTERMEDIATE PROFESSIONAL DEVELOPMENT PERIOD (7-15 years)						12
11							11
10							10
9							9
8			Chief, Audiology/ Hearing Conservation Clinic, Chief Audiologist MEDDAC, Chief, Hearing Conservation, USAEHA, R&D assignment. Exceptional Family Member Program.	AMEDD Officer Adv Course	WORKSHOPS		8
7							7
6							6
5				Language, Airborne, Ranger Training. CAS3	Second Master's in other Health Care fields. Ph.D. (limited number)		5
4	BASIC PROFESSIONAL DEVELOPMENT PERIOD (0-7 years)						4
3		Develop a basic military foundation with emphasis on AMEDD functions. Basic professional knowledge development and performance. Qualify for Certificate of Clinical Competence in Audiology/licensure. Develop leadership skills. Qualify for course Director Council on Accreditation for Hearing Conservation.	Junior position in Auditory Evaluation and Treatment Clinic MEDDAC/MEDCEN, Coordinator, Installation level Hearing Conservation Program, initial positions under supervision of senior certified audiologist.				3
2							2
1					SEMINARS		1
				BASIC AMMEDD OFFICER COURSE			

remain on active duty after their first tour apply for "Voluntary Indefinite" (VI) status. Approximately 50 percent of officers desiring to remain on active duty are selected. Selection for VI status obligates the officers to at least one additional year of active duty. At the end of this period, they may resign their commission. During the basic professional development period opportunities exist as mentioned earlier for continuing military and professional specialty education. Army doctrine defines military education as assimilation of "that body of professional knowledge common to all army officers such as leadership, command, operations, logistics, communication skills, management, etc." Specialty education, on the other hand, encompasses training unique to a particular profession. The basic purpose of formal education beyond the entry level requirement is to prepare the individual for more broad and complex duties. Each level of training, be it military or specialty, should prepare the audiology officer to undertake more responsibility and to achieve a greater sophistication in the specialty. Military courses emphasizing management, leadership and staffing principles are readily available through correspondence courses. Additional academic course work is also encouraged, with the army providing 75 percent of the tuition. Additional specialty training can also be obtained at annual AMEDD audiology short courses, through consultant visits, and by attending professional conventions and seminars.

At some point between the fourth and seventh year on active duty, officers who intend to remain on active duty attend the officer advanced course at Fort Sam Houston. The course provides training in military medical support operations during national emergencies and an overall orientation to staff responsibilities in the Army Medical Department.

Phase 2 of an officer's career is the *intermediate professional development period*, which lasts until the fifteenth year of military service. During this period the audiologist is expected to achieve a high level of specialty proficiency. Additional formal military or civilian training also occurs during this period. Consideration is given for attendance at the Command and General Staff College or the Armed Forces Staff College. Unlike the basic and advanced courses, these courses train officers from all branches of the army. Each program prepares the officer for general duties within field units and as staff officers for larger commands.

A number of audiologists attend Ph.D. programs while on active duty. Each year one or two top applicants are selected for long-term civilian training to obtain doctorate degrees. This opportunity obligates an officer to a minimum of four years on active duty following program completion.

Occupational burnout is always a professional hazard. Alternatives have been provided during the intermediate professional development period to explore alternate health care specialties. For example, education in health care administration may be considered instead of a doctoral program. After completion of the program, the audiologist is awarded a specialty identifier for that area and is eligible for a broader range of military assignments, some outside the original area of specialization.

The third period, which spans the fifteenth through the twenty-third year on active duty is called the *advanced contribution and development period*. The individual now prepares to fill top level management positions, that is, staff or supervisory positions. Emphasis is directed toward executive development by increasing overall knowledge and experience. With the exception of a limited number of officers who attend a senior service college, formal training is on a limited basis. Courses of instruction and assignments are offered outside the specialty area and are directed toward the overall army structure. As the twenty-third year approaches, the *major professional contribution period* begins. During this stage, the army receives its "ultimate dividend" for the education and training provided during earlier career development periods. The officer is now prepared for key leadership positions within the Medical Service Corps. The audiologist, armed with knowledge and expertise in diverse areas, is prepared to direct the planning of major projects and to contribute to long range goals of military audiology within the Army Medical Department.

Civilian Professional Development

The use of civilian health care practitioners may satisfy the overall patient workload, but it also creates additional administrative problems. Military and civilian audiologists, although working in the same environment and performing similar or identical jobs, are managed separately.

Army audiologists have a centralized career management and promotion system. Civilian audiologists and speech-language pathologists, on the other hand, have a decentralized career and promotion system. Civilian staff are generally hired at a fixed grade level and may remain at that level indefinitely. There is little opportunity for career progression, and this is a major cause of professional burnout. This problem is exacerbated by the fact that their military peers are promoted periodically, and eventually outrank them professionally regardless of experience.

The Promotion System

The promotion system for military officers is tied to the four-phase professional development program. Audiologists have the opportunity to be promoted from the entry grade of first lieutenant through the grade of colonel. The various ranks and approximate times for promotion are shown in Table 8-1. Promotions are based on the collective recommendations of a duly appointed board. Promotions are not necessarily considered a reward for past performance. The promotion board also determines if an officer has the credentials and potential to serve at the next higher grade. In this context the officer's entire career and performance record is reviewed. On a best-qualified basis officers are selected for the next higher grade. Officers with less than fourteen years on active duty, who have been considered twice for promotion without success, must resign their commission. In certain cases officers may be offered "selective continuation" for an additional three years. Those with tenure (that is, fourteen years or more service) may be passed over for promotion but are allowed to remain on active duty until they retire. A major may stay on active duty for twenty-two years, a Lieutenant Colonel for twenty-eight years and a Colonel for thirty years. Any officer may retire after twenty years of commissioned service. At that time, retirement pay is 50 percent of base salary. Retirement pay increases 2½ percent per year through 30 years. Thus, officers with 30 years service may retire with 75 percent of their base salary.

PRACTICAL ISSUES IN ADMINISTRATION

Managers have many common administrative responsibilities. The activity must be properly staffed, have a budget to support the program, and have equipment to evaluate and manage the patient. In addition, the program must have a quality assurance program to assure that services are being delivered at an optimum level.

Staffing Requirements

A continual complaint from administrators of military audiology and speech-language pathology programs is that they are understaffed. In general, patient case-loads far exceed staffing requirements. How can an adequate staff be acquired to meet the caseload? Prior to any hiring action, an actual need for additional staff must be determined and documented. Through the use of manpower survey teams, Health Services Command makes the ultimate determination of staffing requirements. The manpower survey team is composed of trained personnel who review the workload of each employee working within a given hospital. Staffing requirements are determined for each hospital by reviewing patient workload and other job responsibilities required of the staff. Table 8-2 illustrates the staffing requirements for audiology services. Even with a standardized audiology workload and mission guide, requirements vary from setting to setting. The army staffing guide handles unique problems with a "local appraisal." This appraisal allows the manager to document the special functions not contained in the staffing guide. Speech language services, for instance, are always reviewed by "local appraisal."

If new functions should emerge between manpower surveys, scheduled approximately at three-year intervals, a "schedule X" may be submitted to substantiate an additional position to cover the new workload. This schedule is sent through administrative hospital channels to the Health Services Command. Based on data provided in the schedule, increased manpower needs may be approved, although a recommendation for reduced staff may also result.

Unfortunately, existing requirements do not guarantee that additional staff will be hired to meet the workload. Requirements almost always exceed the authorized number of employees available to do the job. For example, there is a recognized requirement for eighty-eight Army audiologists to meet the clinical and hearing conservation needs of the army. The number of authorized audiologists is only 71 percent of the recognized requirements. To complicate matters, Congress has imposed a ceiling on the total number of officers allowed in the army. No

TABLE 8-2   Manpower Guide for Army Audiology and Speech-Language Pathology Services

MANPOWER GUIDE FOR ARMY AUDIOLOGY AND SPEECH-LANGUAGE PATHOLOGY SERVICES

Work Performed: Conducts quantitative audiological examinations and evaluations of auditory pathways.
Prescribes and implements non-medical treatment to conserve or improve communication ability. Designs, develops and maintains the Hearing Conservation Program, counsels patients about hearing problems. Makes ear mold impressions for hearing aid users and fits issues hearing protective devices. Performs audiometric screenings.

Yardstick	Population supported (thousands)	6	15	24	33
	Manpower requirement	2	3	4	5
	Interval Rate	·.111	.111	.111	

	Military positions				Position delineation	Number of positions				Civilian positions	
Line	Duty position title	BR	MOS Code	Grade						Job Title	Code
1	AUDIOLOGIST	MS	68M	LTC/MAJ	C	···	···	1	1	AUDIOLOGIST	GS-0665
2	AUDIOLOGIST	MS	68M	CPT/LT	C	1	1	1	1	AUDIOLOGIST	GS-0665
3	ENT SPECIALIST	···	91U20	E5	C	···	···	···	1	HEALTH TECHNICIAN	GS-0665
4	ENT SPECIALIST	···	91U10	E4	C	1	1	1	1	HEALTH TECHNICIAN	GS-0665
5	ENT SPECIALIST	···	91U10	E3	C	···	1	1	1	HEALTH TECHNICIAN	GS-0665
6	CLERK TYPIST	···	71L10	E3	C	···	···	···	···	CLERK TYPIST	GS-0665

FOOTNOTES:
Installation military population.
Where Audiology is not collocated with another clinic or where an Administrative Support Division has not been established, clerical support, when required, will be determined by local appraisal.
Note 1: When determining MEDCEN staffing, local appraisal based on quantitative time/task workload data must be considered for the following additional responsibilities:
Hearing Aid Evaluation, consultation, issue and repair
Electronystagmography (ENG)
Auditory Brainstem Evoke Response (ABR)
Note 2: Reception station coverage will be determined through local appraisal.
Note 3: Speech Pathology requirements will be determined by local appraisal through time/task documentation (i.e., diagnostic evaluations, therapy visits, administration and consultations).
Note 4: To permit development of a more definitive yardstick, time/task data for clinic visits and the Hearing Conservation Program for both audiologists and technicians should be documented on Schedules X.
Note 5: The number of personnel (both military and civilian) working in noise hazardous areas must be documented on Schedule X.

matter how necessary the requirement, creating a new authorization for an additional army audiologist would result in the elimination of an officer from some other specialty. In order to meet the existing workload without an increase in officers, each hospital has funding to hire civilians. Depending on the overall hospital budget for civilian payrolls, a given number of audiologists and speech-language pathologists can be hired. Even with the combination of military and civilian staff, authorizations rarely match requirements. To compensate for the gap in requirement and authorization levels, technicians often assist the audiologist in clinical and hearing conservation programs. Duties may include supervised audiometric testing, taking of earmold impressions for hearing aid fittings, fitting and issuing hearing protective devices, electronystagmography, and various record-keeping responsibilities. Military audiology technicians who are enlisted hospital corpsmen receive eighteen weeks of didactic and on-the-job training prior to being assigned to an audiology facility.

Budget

A misconception often exists in socialized health care systems that budgetary matters are not really a problem. While revenue is not generated from fees per service, the overall budget is directly tied to the number of patient contacts, staff salaries, equipment, supplies, and costs for continuing education. The Army Medical Department receives a share of the overall defense budget. In turn each medical command receives funds to operate facilities under its jurisdiction. The overall budget is broken into several separate funds. Individual budgets are maintained for major construction projects, major equipment purchases, staff salaries, consumable clinic supplies, etc. An efficiently managed facility is rewarded with a realistic operating budget. To receive funds that adequately cover the overall costs of operating a service the administrator must maintain adequate documentation for use in manpower surveys. In addition, supportive personnel in nontechnical positions can be used to hold the overall salaries within the operating budget. Other administrative measures must also be dealt with in an efficient manner. Timely submission of administrative workload reports, controlling the use of sick leave and overtime, and other conscientious efforts to curb waste are a constant concern in socialized health care systems and in government.

Equipment

The administrator must intensively manage the clinic's equipment procurement program. The purchasing of new equipment and replacement of obsolete items to support clinical audiology and hearing conservation programs are determined by centralized guidelines. There are three separate programs under which equipment can be purchased: the Medical Care Support Equipment (MEDCASE) Program, the Capital Expense Equipment Program (CEEP), and the annual supply budget.

The MEDCASE program supports medical activities' needs for equipment over a five-year period. The system is designed for items over $3,000 and permits advance planning for equipment needs for new facilities, program expansions, state-of-the-art advances and other anticipated needs. The manager must annually update each year in the five-year plan to ensure that present and future requests are valid.

Replacement equipment cannot be requested without extensive documentation from maintenance personnel. A centrally managed repair record must accompany requests for new equipment to replace existing equipment. Equipment cannot be replaced solely on the basis of age. When documented maintenance costs exceed the equipment's present value, new equipment is authorized with the maintenance record providing objective evidence of need.

Often, however, total hospital MEDCASE requirements exceed the existing authorized budget. Service chiefs from each hospital department meet to prioritize all equipment needs on a rank order basis. Items prioritized from number one downward are purchased until funds are exhausted. Items that are not purchased are carried over to the next fiscal year. Obviously this can delay purchases in the subsequent year's budget.

MEDCASE requests are approved by a centralized agency within the Army Medical Department. Requests for equipment in each specialty area are forwarded to the appropriate consultant for review. Equipment requests are approved if a valid requirement for the item is perceived and if there is physical space to house the equipment, and staff to operate it. Determinations must also be made that new equipment can be maintained, and that old equipment has reached its life expectancy. The item must also be purchased on a competitive bid basis.

The CEEP program is designed for purchases of equipment ranging from $1,000 to $2,999 in value. Requests are submitted annually. They are prioritized and purchased according to rank order. Strong clinical justifications (as well as lobbying efforts by the administrator) are major determinants in prioritization of equipment needs. A third source for equipment with small dollar value is the supply budget. This budget is managed by program directors at their discretion and can be used to purchase small cost items.

An often underutilized vehicle for equipment procurement is through hospitals' clinical investigation departments. When an area of research is acceptable to the hospital but requires additional equipment, the Clinical Investigations Service may provide the funding. The equipment generally becomes the property of the clinic conducting the research.

Hearing Aids

The army purchases hearing aids through a contract with the Veterans Administration. There are several advantages in purchasing hearing aids through this procedure. Army audiologists are allowed to participate in the annual Veterans Administration hearing aid selection program (described in Dr. Spuehler's chapter). This selection and purchasing system keeps management costs to a minimum and provides only top quality hearing aids that meet rigorous laboratory quality standards. Due to the large quantity of hearing aids purchased—the army purchased 13,000 in fiscal year 1986 and this amount is increasing at a rate of approximately 10 percent annually—the price per unit is low with each company providing a full two-year warranty. The number of different models in use by the army is also kept to a minimum. Intensive management of hearing aids facilitates a centralized issuing system within each health service region and facilitates the centralized army hearing aid repair program.

Quality Assurance in the Delivery of Speech Language and Hearing Services in the Army

Quality assurance is an essential factor in determining the success of speech-language and hearing programs. There are several measures of quality assurance. The three areas that focus on speech-language and hearing in the army concern (1) individual certification, (2) institutional accreditation and (3) continuing education. Certification/state licensure for audiologists and speech language pathologists, both military and civilian, became mandatory in 1985. Mandatory certification was enacted to ensure that all health care providers met minimal nationally accepted professional standards, and to provide a vehicle for credentialing all health care providers in army health care facilities.

Army audiologists are required to obtain their Certification of Clinical Competence during their initial three years of active duty. If certification is not gained the officer may be asked to leave the army.

Although not mandatory, accreditation as a hearing conservation course director is highly desirable for all audiology officers. This accreditation is offered by the Council on Accreditation of Occupational Hearing Conservation. Audiologists can then in turn offer certification courses to other employees or technicians at their local post. This program eliminates the need to send new employees to civilian programs, often at considerable expense and time lost from the job.

Institutional accreditation by the Professional Standards Board at ASHA is actively encouraged for speech-language and hearing services in army hospitals. Most medical centers have or are in the process of making application for PSB accreditation. Such accreditation requests are warmly encouraged by the local hospital administration as the Joint Commission on Accreditation of Hospitals (JCAH) views this as a strong hospital quality assurance measure.

BENEFICIARIES OF ARMY HEALTH CARE

Socialized health care has restrictions on the categories of patients that may be offered service. In addition, those necessary services not available must have a backup system in order that proper treatment is given. The army has two systems, one for health care outside of the military, and the other system to ensure that proper facilities are available for those patients in need. This section will discuss patient eligibility, civilian health care and the exceptional family member program.

Patients Eligible for Care

Some confusion exists about eligibility for health care from the military and the Veterans Administration (VA). In most cases, the medical systems and patient populations are separate and distinct. Active duty personnel and their dependents are eligible for military health care as are retired military personnel and their dependents. There are other categories of eligible personnel that may be designated as health care beneficiaries by the Department of the Army, such as members of the diplomatic corps and foreign military personnel. VA medical facilities do not treat active duty personnel or their dependents. Veterans (discharged or retired) with a service-connected disability are alone eligible for VA health benefits. Retired personnel and their dependents without a service-connected disability are not eligible for care. A person may be eligible for care from both systems when the individual has retired from the military and has established a service-connected disability with the VA. In this special case, retired service members who have service-connected hearing loss are eligible for care in either, or both, programs.

Civilian Health and Medical Program
of the Uniformed Services

The army health care system has provisions to cover the costs for medical services not available at a given hospital. The system is similar to insurance programs in which a certain deductible must be borne by the patient. People who are eligible for medical care in the army are also eligible for care under the Civilian Health and Medical Program of the Uniformed Services (CHAMPUS) when specific medical treatment cannot be provided by the local medical facility. Certain speech-language and audiology services are covered by the CHAMPUS program for the handicapped. Under the program the sponsor pays an initial share of the monthly cost according to his or her pay grade and the government pays an amount not to exceed a maximum of $1,000 monthly. As with third party payments in the civilian sector, cumbersome restrictions apply to speech and hearing services. All care must be prescribed by a physician and the services must be rendered as part of the treatment of a physical defect rather than as an educational or training deficit. The initial claim submitted for a course of speech-language therapy must include a signed prescription/statement from the attending physician indicating: (1) complete medical diagnosis and date of onset; (2) number of speech therapy sessions per week and length of therapy sessions; (3) established length of time services will be required; (4) the short-term and long-term goals of the program; and (5) that a progress report will be provided by the speech pathologist to the attending physician at the thirtieth therapy session. CHAMPUS will not cover speech therapy provided to any child who is eligible to receive therapy through the public school system, the state of residence, or another federal agency.

CHAMPUS allows purchasing of hearing aids. Minimal medical and audiometric criteria must be satisfied (see appendix 2) and the audiologic examination must have been conducted or supervised by an audiologist. Active duty dependents of all ages are eligible for amplification. CHAMPUS will generally approve the purchase of hearing aids (monaural or binaural fittings) when in the professional opinion of the audiologist or physician, amplification is warranted.

Exceptional Family Member Program

The Army Medical Department has the responsibility for identifying and coding the special education and health needs of family members of army personnel and forwarding this information to the army assignments branch. This information aids the army in selecting assignments for military personnel where the special educational needs of their dependents can be accommodated. Speech-language pathology and audiology services are an important aspect of the program.

Medical teams provide the evaluation and coding services for identifying family members with potential special education needs. Exceptional Family Member teams provide input to the exceptional family member's individual development plan in coordination with the Department of Defense School System. Thus, the medical aspects of speech-language hearing problems are closely coordinated with the child's educational needs.

The typical Exceptional Family Member team consists of the following members: the director, a developmental pediatrician, a social worker, child psychologist, psychometrician, occupational therapist, physical therapist, OT technician, audiologist, speech-language pathologist, public health nurse, and administrative support. The team evaluates, staffs and coordinates the special education needs of each child on a case-by-case basis. A single team member assumes responsibility for management of each case and becomes in essence the team leader for that child and family. In Europe, speech and language problems represent the second most common handicapping condition among school-age military dependents.

Administrative support for each team is given through the hospital facility to which the team is attached. To ensure the integrity of the team, however, staff and equipment are separated from the hospital facility.

SUGGESTIONS FOR FUTURE ADMINISTRATORS OF ARMY SPEECH-LANGUAGE AND HEARING PROGRAMS

Administrators of speech-language and hearing services in the military will see an increasing number of women entering the military. With the federal deficit reaching record-breaking figures cost containment will affect every health care program in the government. This section will discuss these important issues.

Women Audiology Officers

Army audiology officers are not exclusively male. For the past five years the ratio of applications for direct commission of women to men has been approximately 60/40. Nevertheless, the upward trend of women on active duty has not paralleled the growth of women in the profession of audiology. The 1983 ASHA data base (Fein, 1984) suggests that only 7½ percent of graduates from speech-language pathology and audiology programs are males. Sixty-five percent of the audiologists possessing the Certificate of Clinical Competence are females. The percentage of women in the field continues to increase. Although the total number of female audiologists in the army is much lower than in other employment settings there has been a dramatic increase in the percentage since 1969. In that year the first woman received a commission. It was another eight years before a second woman received a commission. From two female officers in 1977 (see fig. 8–3) the number increased to six in 1980 and by 1985 there were fifteen. By 1988 over 30 percent and by 1992 half of the army audiology officers will be women. As knowledge of the employment setting and career benefits increase, and the overall stigma of the military as a male-dominated organization declines, more and more women will find the service a viable career option.

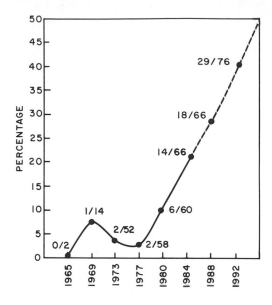

FIGURE 8-3 Proportion of Female to Total Army Audiology Officers Beginning in 1965.

Cost Containment

The federal government has several health care programs that tend to duplicate each other. Each branch of the military, the Veterans Administration and other smaller programs offer speech and hearing services. In most cases patients are restricted to only one health care system. As a cost-saving measure future administrators should seek ways to break down system barriers. Creation of a health care system which allows reciprocal treatment for classes of patients, for example, could eliminate duplicate services within a geographical area.

Administrators of army programs may wish to explore the purchase of high volume items from an army-based procurement program. The VA system has been of great benefit to the military in supplying hearing aids. However, the present volume might be more efficiently handled through direct purchasing, thereby eliminating the middleman.

The issue of civilian job satisfaction must always be on the mind of the military administrator. While the thrust is toward career progression of military officers, the civilian workforce provides the consistency and continuity of the majority of the hearing and speech programs. Continuing efforts must be made to create job satisfaction and career enhancement for the civilian staff.

SUMMARY

The army's speech-language and hearing programs offer a view of a centralized model of health care. From management of individual career planning to administration of health care facilities, a centrally based management model exists within the Army Medical Department. The roots of the army's audiology program extend back to the World War II rehabilitation program. Today, as much emphasis is placed on prevention as on diagnosis, treatment and rehabilitation. It is anticipated that the demand for the speech and hearing services in the army will continue to grow and will serve as a model for speech and hearing services for the civilian community.

REFERENCES

AMERICAN SPEECH-LANGUAGE HEARING ASSOCIATION EDITORIAL STAFF. (1967). "MOS 3360," *Asha*, 9, 11.

BERRY G. (1942). "Reeducation of the deafened soldier, in ophthalmology and otolaryngology," *Military Service Manuals*, ed. Subcommittee on Division of Medical Sciences of the National Research Council. Philadelphia: W. B. Saunders Co., 257.

CANFIELD, N. (1957). "Administrative aspects of otolaryngology," in *Surgery in World War II: Ophthalmology and Otolaryngology*, ed. N. Canfield. Washington D.C.: U.S. Government Printing Office.

CANFIELD, N. AND L. MORRISETT. (1947). "Military aural rehabilitation," in *Hearing and Deafness: A Guide for Laymen*, ed H. Davis. New York, NY: Murray Hill Books, Inc.

FEIN, D. (1984). "Vive la difference," *Asha*, 26, 35.

MORRISSETT, L. (1957). "The aural rehabilitation program for the deafened and hard of hearing," in *Surgery in World War II: Ophthalmology and Otolaryngology*, ed. N. Canfield. Washington, D.C.: U.S. Government Printing Office.

NORTHERN, JERRY L. AND J. ENDICOTT. (1968). "Military opportunities in speech pathology and audiology," *Asha, 10*, 325–330.

WALDEN, B., R. PROSEK, AND D. WORTHINGTON. (1975). *The Prevalence of Hearing Loss within Selected U.S. Army Branches*, Washington, D.C.: Army Medical Research and Development Command, Interagency No. 1AO 4745.

9 The Veterans' Administration Program in Speech Pathology and Audiology

Henry E. Spuehler*

INTRODUCTION

A frequently heard saying within the Veterans Administration is that once you have seen one VA medical center, you have seen one medical center. The saying attempts to stress the fact that, although the Veterans Administration is thought to be a unified federal agency, there are significant differences among the VA medical centers. The primary reason for these differences lies in the sizes of the medical centers and the range of patient services that can be provided. For example, sophisticated surgical or radiology services might only be provided in a larger VA medical center.

In an attempt to provide veterans with all the patient services that might be needed, the VA has grouped medical centers into medical districts. Each medical district has a cross-section of different-sized medical centers. If open heart surgery is needed for a veteran, he may be sent to a larger medical center within the district where the operation can be conducted.

The audiology and speech pathology programs within the VA are also affected by the VA medical center differences. There is not, nor will there be in the future, an audiology and speech pathology program in each of the medical centers. There are medical centers that are too small to support such a program and, like other

---

*Dr. Spuehler is director, Audiology and Speech Pathology Service, Veteran's Administration Central Office, Washington, D.C.

programs in a specific facility, it might be necessary for the veteran to be transported to another medical center within the district for evaluation and/or treatment of a speech or hearing disorder. In some instances, a staff audiologist or speech pathologist may also be detailed to travel to a smaller medical center on a periodic basis to provide the needed assistance.

When the VA audiology and speech pathology program is compared to similar programs both inside and outside the federal sector, it would appear that there are many aspects of the VA program that are more appealing to audiologists and speech pathologists seeking professional employment. These position advantages will be described later, but a brief overview of the growth of audiology and speech pathology within the VA might assist in illustrating how they evolved.

VA Audiology and Speech Pathology
Program Background

Historically, the VA Audiology and Speech Pathology program originated within the aural rehabilitation program of the armed forces that was established in World War II. A previous chapter described these programs and there is no need to discuss the goals or purposes of the military aural rehabilitation programs again. When World War II came to an end, it became clear that the Veterans Administration would be responsible for the care of all those individuals who had been patients in the military aural rehabilitation centers, as well as all other veterans who had incurred services connected hearing impairments. As can be seen, the impetus for establishing a program within the VA was the audiological needs of the veterans.

In 1945, Dr. Norton Canfield, an otolaryngologist from Yale University School of Medicine, was appointed a consultant to the chief medical director of the Veterans Administration for the purpose of establishing services for veterans with aural handicaps, similar to the services that had been available during wartime in the aural rehabilitation centers. Dr. Canfield established what was known as audiology and speech correction services under a division of VA called Medical Rehabilitation Service, later to be called the Physical Medicine and Rehabilitation Service, and now known as the Rehabilitation Medicine Service.

Although the program at that time was called audiology and speech correction, the provision of speech pathology services was divided. Aphasia and what were considered psychogenic speech disorders were the responsibility of the Psychiatry and Neurology Service. Voice and articulation problems associated with organic conditions, and speech problems related to hearing impairments, were the responsibility of the Medical Rehabilitation Service. This division of speech disorders remained until the early 1960s, when they were combined under a chief of Audiology and Speech Pathology.

In 1946, Edward H. Truex, Jr., M.D. was employed on a part-time basis to manage the audiology and speech correction program. Following Dr. Truex, Aram Glorig, M.D. and Merle Ansberry, Ph.D. were employed by the VA to manage the program. Dr. Ansberry, was the first full-time employee in audiology and speech correction in Central Office. Kenneth O. Johnson, Ph.D. was chief from 1954 to 1956, Bernard Anderman, Ed.D. was chief from 1956 to 1980. It should be mentioned that since the appointment of Dr. Kenneth O. Johnson, the chief of the program has been an individual who has had experience within the VA before assuming the position.

VA Audiology Review Program

It will become evident to the readers of this chapter that the Audiology and Speech Pathology program has achieved a professional status within the agency that is found only in very few other organizations. One of the primary reasons that the status was achieved was the establishment of the ten-year review of veterans who were receiving compensation for hearing impairment and had received their hearing compensation examinations prior to 1954.

Shortly after Dr. Kenneth O. Johnson was employed as the Central Office chief of Audiology and Speech Pathology, he convinced the administrator of the VA that there was a significant number of veterans who were receiving compensation that was based upon little more than a "watch tick" or "whispered voice" test, and that these test results were probably highly unreliable. Dr. Johnson convinced the VA that a review program should be established in 1955 to reevaluate all veterans who were receiving compensation for a hearing impairment prior to that time. The audiology review program was conducted over a ten-year period and approximately 100,000 veterans were reevaluated for their organic hearing acuity.

The results of the review program made the audiology program very popular and visible within the VA system. An analysis conducted on the first 25,000 veterans reevaluated produced a yearly saving in compensation of approximately $15 million. By the end of the audiology review program, this annual compensation savings statistic increased almost threefold. With this type of cost saving, it is very easy to see why the audiology program rapidly became highly esteemed within the VA.

The VA audiology review program influenced more than just a cost-saving procedure for the VA. A direct result of this program was the establishment of high standards of professionalism for audiologists and the field of audiology in programs both within and outside the federal government. Many of the audiological procedures currently being used in the field at that time were developed in the VA. VA-trained audiologists were in demand throughout the nation, and the VA program still has the reputation of training and employing highly competent audiologists.

VA Hearing Aid Distribution Program

From the time that audiology and speech pathology services were offered in the VA, the provision of hearing aids to eligible veterans has been an integral part of the program. Immediately after World War II, veterans were sent to hearing aid dealers for their needed instruments. As the number of VA audiology programs grew, procedures were developed to provide the veterans their hearing aids directly through the VA. The current nationwide hearing aid distribution program has been developed over a period of more than thirty years and is heralded internationally as an excellent system.

The most distinctive feature of the VA hearing aid distribution program is that the veteran is issued the hearing aid that provides him or her the most satisfaction. It is a recognized fact that, although two hearing aids might be of the same manufacturer make and model, there can be a slight difference in the electroacoustic characteristics of the two aids that will result in a quality difference noted by a hearing aid wearer.

Each year, the VA invites hearing aid manufacturers nationwide to submit models of their instruments for contract consideration. For each manufacturer responding positively, the VA facility closest to the manufacturer sends a representative of Supply Service to the company and has him or her randomly choose three hearing aids of the make and model that are to be considered. All of the hearing aids submitted are then sent to the National Bureau of Standards for analysis. Since 1955, the VA has contracted with the National Bureau of Standards to conduct tests of the electronacoustic characteristics of all hearing aids that are submitted. The results of these tests are forwarded to the VA for their contractual consideration.

For the past thirty years, a consultant group of audiologists from both within and outside the VA has been convened annually to determine which of the hearing aids submitted each year will be placed on the following year's contract. The group is composed of audiologists who are continually active in clinical settings and bring to the meeting their experience working with a variety of hearing aid instruments with a large number of patients. The consultant group reviews the hearing aid needs of the VA for the coming year when considering which aids will be on contract. The price of the hearing aid is rarely used as a selection criterion in this process.

After the hearing aids have been selected by the consultant group, contracts are made with each manufacturer and, for each new contract year, hearing aids are purchased from the manufacturers by the VA Prosthetics Distribution Center (PDC) in Denver for nationwide distribution to the current fifty-four VA locations where hearing aids are stocked. When a hearing aid is issued to a veteran, the audiology clinic requests a replacement of the hearing aid from the PDC. The current time involved in replacing a hearing aid is approximately a week to ten days. There are efforts being made to shorten this replacement time to four days in the near future. Therefore, all hearing aids within the VA are purchased and replaced by the PDC and the budget for purchasing hearing aids and hearing aid batteries is controlled at that one location.

Hearing aids are issued only to those veterans who have eligibility as defined by congressional legislation. Eligibility for these services will be discussed later in this chapter but it should be noted that, for the majority of the veterans receiving a hearing aid, the hearing aid, batteries and care or repair are all provided free by the VA. When the veteran needs to have a hearing aid repaired or needs batteries, the hearing aid or the request for batteries is sent directly to the PDC by the veteran. The turnaround time for these requests is also minimal.

During fiscal year 1984, more than 44,000 hearing aids were issued through the VA system. The cost to the VA for the purchase of the needed hearing aids and batteries was close to $7 million. When the total cost of the program is given, it would appear that it is extremely expensive. Actually, it is probably one of the most cost-effective programs in government. Several congressional investigations of the VA national hearing aid program have been conducted over the last ten years. These investigations have been motivated by reports that it costs the VA $700 to $1000 for each hearing aid a veteran receives. The results of the congressional investigations showed that this was a gross overestimate. The most recent analysis of the VA hearing aid program showed that the average cost of issuing a hearing aid to a veteran was $239. This average-cost statistic includes the cost of the hearing aid to the VA plus the cost of the otologic and audiologic examinations, the provision of hearing aid orientation, earmold fabrication, cost of hearing aid batteries for a one-year period, cost of paperwork processing, beneficiary travel expenses for the veteran, the overhead costs of the medical center, and the cost of the contract with the National Bureau of Standards. When the $7 million dollar program is now reexamined from the perspective of cost per hearing aid, the program can be shown to be extremely cost-effective. It is no wonder that the VA hearing aid distribution program is heralded internationally.

VA Central Office Organizational Development

The organizational development of the Central Office program of the VA Audiology and Speech Pathology program differed slightly from that of programs in the medical centers. As mentioned previously, the Central Office program was originally placed under the Medical Rehabilitation Service. After that it was placed under the Outpatient Service, the Extended Care Service, and then back to the Medical Rehabilitation Service, which was then known as just the Rehabilitation Service. In 1980, the Audiology and Speech Pathology program was finally designated as a separate service.

VA Agency Organizational Structure

To better understand where the audiology and speech pathology program is placed within the total agency, the overall Veterans Administration agency should be briefly described.

The VA has three major divisions. One division is called the Department of Memorial Affairs (DMA) which has the responsibility of developing, monitoring and planning cemeteries and/or monuments for veterans. A second division is the Department of Veterans Benefits (DVB) that is responsible for the payment of veterans' compensation, the GI Bill program, housing loans and veterans' insurance programs. The third division is the Department of Medicine and Surgery (DM&S) which has the responsibility of veteran patient care.

The head of the VA agency is known as the administrator and is appointed by the president. Each of the three divisions has a director appointed by Congress. The director of the Department of Medicine and Surgery is known as the chief medical director and is always a physician. Within DM&S, there are eight assistants to the director known as assistant chief medical directors (ACMDs), and one of these individuals is the ACMD for Professional Services. The Audiology and Speech Pathology Service is placed under this ACMD within Central Office.

VA Medical Center Organizational Development

In the VA medical centers, the majority of the programs achieved a service status much more easily than did Central Office. If the program is started at a medical center with only one professional, that individual is usually placed under an existing service for at least administrative purposes. Once a program has employed at least two full-time professionals, it may be raised to a service level though a recommendation by the medical center director.

It should be noted that, within the VA medical centers, the overall organizational structure is primarily dependent upon the type of services that are performed. The medical center director will have an associate medical center director to manage the administrative services. If the center is large, there will probably be both an associate and an assistant medical center director. Professional services are placed under the chief of staff, who is always a physician. Each professional service has a chief and, if the staff is large, there can be sections and even units within the service. The majority of the audiology and speech pathology programs within the VA are designated as services and are directly under the medical center chief of staff. The advantages of this type of organizational placement will be described in more detail later, but when it is realized that the chief of the Audiology and Speech Pathology Service within the VA has the same organizational placement as the chief of Surgery or the chief of Medicine, the implications for administration, planning and development are tremendous.

THE SPEECH-LANGUAGE-HEARING PROGRAM IN A VA MEDICAL CENTER SETTING

The introduction of this chapter has attempted to provide an overview of the general structure of the VA Audiology and Speech Pathology program both within Central Office and at the local medical centers. The remaining sections of this chapter will concentrate more on the dynamics of the local medical centers with minor references to the responsibilities of the Central Office director. The Veterans Administration, like many other federal agencies, has delegated the authority of local program planning to the medical center service chiefs, while the program official in Central Office does professional planning.

The chief and the staff of an audiology and speech pathology service in a VA medical center must be constantly aware of the fact that their service functions as a referral program. Their existence is based upon their ability to obtain referrals from either the "bed" services or the outpatient service of that medical center. No veteran patient is ever considered to be exclusively theirs. The veteran patients are always the responsibility of a primary physician. Therefore, the capability of each staff audiologist and/or speech pathologist to be productive is directly related to the reputation the program has with the medical center physicians. It is possible to have an excellent staff and outstanding facilities, but if no veteran patients are referred there will be no program.

VA MEDICAL CENTER MISSION GUIDELINES

Each of the professional and administrative services within the medical center must actively promote the overall mission of the local medical center as well as the mission of the Veterans Administration agency. Within the VA Department of Medicine and Surgery, the mission of all medical centers is to (1) provide quality patient care; (2) participate in the training of medical care professionals; (3) conduct meaningful research; and (4) coordinate VA medical care activities with community programs. The audiology and speech pathology service in each medical center is obligated to develop clinical and administrative policies and procedures for the service that will outline exactly how the service intends to accomplish its responsibility in achieving the medical center mission.

In addition to the overall mission of the VA, annual mission statements are announced by the chief medical director and it becomes the responsibility of the service chiefs to assist the medical center in providing action plans that will answer the needs of these annual mission statements. For example, if the chief medical director issues a mission statement that outlines the need for developing quality medical care for the aging veteran, the service chiefs are to provide the medical center with action plans that will outline what and how these needs will be addressed in the coming year. Mission statements from the chief medical director can change from year to year but the overall mission of the VA always remains the same.

AUDIOLOGY AND SPEECH PATHOLOGY ORGANIZATIONAL PLACEMENT

As was mentioned previously, the typical organization placement for the chief of the audiology and speech pathology program is directly under the medical center's chief of staff. All administrative problems and reports are directed to the chief of staff for his or her final decision and possible signature. The administrative problems forwarded by the chief are usually associated with space, staff, or money, and must be directed through the chief of staff for his or her information so that overall planning for the professional services wihin the medical center can be effectively conducted.

There is a secondary organizational placement that also exists for the service chief. All service chiefs in the VA Department of Medicine and Surgery are classified within what is called a centralized position. When a vacancy for a service chief exists, the medical center must contact the program official in Central Office to ask for assistance in filling the vacancy. The program official announces the position nationwide within the VA and the responses that are obtained are reviewed before they are sent to the medical center director and chief of staff. The selection of the service chief is then made jointly by Central Office and the local medical center from the candidates who have applied for the position. If it is decided that the candidates are not of high enough quality, the program official must provide additional candidates until a final decision is reached. Because the selection of the service chief has been made through the Central Office program official, the position is labeled as being *centralized*.

The rationale for having service chief positions centralized is based upon a need for nationwide continuity in these positions. Although the funds to employ the individual in the centralized position are at the local medical center, there is a nationwide effort to make each service similar to all others in other medical centers. The medical center service chief, therefore, has a dual responsibility in the VA. The chief's first responsibility is directly to the local medical center, while the second responsibility is to the program official at Central Office.

There are advantages in being in a centralized program. The Central Office program official can be contacted directly by the medical center service chief for professional and, in some instances, administrative assistance. There are many instances when opportunities arise for the distribution of additional staff, funds or even equipment for Central Office and, because the medical center chief is an indirect responsibility of the Central Office official, direct distribution of these resources can be made. If the chief were only responsible to the medical center, there would be no way that resources could be made available from Central Office.

Another advantage of being in a centralized position is that the service chief is given added job security. The centralized service chief cannot be forced to resign through a decision by the medical center director or chief of staff. Any such adverse action leveled at the person in a centralized position can be accomplished only with the approval of the Central Office program official. Although these types of personnel actions occur very infrequently, it is heartening for the service chief to know that job security does exist. There have been instances where the chief of staff and a service chief have experienced personality conflicts. When this has happened, the CO program official has been requested to make a visit to help resolve the problems. If the service chief were not centralized, this outside assistance would not be available.

Therefore, the chief of the audiology and speech pathology service will report directly to the chief of staff for the majority of administrative problems and, in some instances, will also be reporting to the program official in Central Office for some administrative or even professional assistance.

Within the area associated with medical center professional problems, the chief of audiology and speech pathology is generally able to communicate directly with other service chiefs or medical center staff without needing to go through the chief of staff. The placement of the service directly under the chief of staff allows the chief to go laterally within the organization to resolve problems. If there is a problem with the management of a patient, the service chief can contact the physician in charge of the patient to effect a solution. In some medical centers, service chiefs are also given the authority of referral. This allows the audiology and speech pathology chief the ability to refer a patient to another medical center service for needed assistance. Of course, if such a referral were to be made, the physician in charge of the patient would be made aware of the recommendation.

VA audiologists and speech pathologists have the reputation of being professionals within their field. They are the sole authority for the evaluation and treatment of speech, language and hearing disorders and have the responsibility of providing the veteran patients with what is needed to obtain quality care. If a part of the audiology evaluation indicates that a thorough neurological examination should be conducted, the responsibility of making that referral is carried by the audiologist. Referrals to audiology and speech pathology are made in general terms. A typical referral to speech pathology would be to evaluate the patient's inability to communicate. It is then up to the speech pathologist to determine what type of evaluation should be conducted and make the appropriate recommendation to ensure that the patient will ultimately receive quality care.

STAFFING CRITERIA FOR MEDICAL CENTER PROGRAMS

When discussing the role of audiologists and/or speech pathologists within the Veterans Administration programs, it should be noted that staffing criteria have been developed to assist local medical centers and the program official in CO to determine the professional needs for any program. As with any other criteria, these staffing standards are only guidelines and, for planning purposes, have been conservatively developed. With the incidence of communication problems among aging veteran patients increasing significantly, it would be overwhelming to some medical centers to realize the number of audiologists and/or speech pathologists that would be needed to meet patient needs. For this reason, the staffing criteria are considered conservative estimates with the hope that, once an audiology and speech pathology program is established at a medical center, future needs will become apparent from the workload that is generated.

VA staffing criteria for speech pathologists and audiologists specify one speech pathologist for every 200 general medical or surgical beds, every 250 domiciliary beds, every 60 nursing home care unit beds, and every 500 neuropsychiatric beds. There should be one audiologist for every two speech pathologists in a medical center with a small outpatient workload and in medical centers where there is no large demand for hearing aid evaluations or compensation examinations. Where a hearing aid evaluation and compensation examination program has been authorized by Central Office, additional audiologists will be necessary. The exact number of audiologists that will be needed is determined by the CO program official.

SPACE CRITERIA FOR MEDICAL CENTER PROGRAMS

Criteria for the audiology and speech pathology service space have also been developed over a period of years. There are two general types of audiology and speech pathology programs within the VA. The first is classified as a *basic program* and is capable of conducting all audiology and speech pathology services except very sophisticated types of audiological procedures, hearing aid evaluations, and audiology compensation examinations. The basic program is typically found in the smaller medical centers. If veterans need audiology and/or speech pathology services that are not available in a basic program, they are referred to the closest medical center capable of providing the needed evaluation and/or treatment.

The second type of program is an *extended program.* All professionally known audiology and speech pathology procedures are available in an extended program. The space criteria for the extended programs includes the following:

Audiology and Speech Pathology Space Criteria

FUNCTION	SQ. FT.
OFFICES	
Chief of service	150
Professional staff	140 each
Secretary	120
Clerks	90 each
Trainees	70 each
CLINICAL AREA	
Waiting room	200
Prefabricated sound suite	
(one sound suite for each audiologist	
plus one if a training program exists)	260 each
Speech pathology group therapy	225
Aural rehabilitation	300
Instrument calibration	200
Acoustic impedance	120
Electronystagmography	130
Earmold fabrication	120
RESEARCH AREA	
Resarch space as needed for audiology	
and/or speech pathology	

PATIENT MIX WITHIN MEDICAL CENTER PROGRAMS

Only veterans who are determined eligible are provided audiology and/or speech pathology services. This eligibility must be established prior to the time that the service is given. Eligibility has been mandated by congressional legislation and is established within the medical center by the staff of the Medical Administration Service.

Veterans who have a service-connected hearing or, very rarely, a speech impairment are eligible for audiology and/or speech pathology services at any time. Currently, veterans who are receiving 50 percent compensation for any service-connected disorder, World War I veterans, and POWs are also considered eligible for audiology and speech pathology services. In addition, any hospitalized veteran or veteran on a continuing outpatient status can receive assistance from our program. Except for the last group, all the other veterans mentioned are considered eligible for hearing aids also. Hospitalized veterans and veterans on a continuing outpatient status can receive a hearing aid if their hearing impairments are serious enough to interfere with their receiving proper medical treatment. It should also be mentioned that all veterans seen in an audiology and speech pathology program must be referred through a physician. If the veteran is an inpatient, he or she will be referred by the physician in charge of the ward. Outpatients are referred by the chief of the outpatient service and, in the case of audiology referrals, must be seen by an ENT physician before being sent to audiology.

The types of patients referred to the audiology and speech pathology service will vary somewhat according to the size of the medical center. Obviously, if the medical center has a limited neurology service or just a part-time ENT physician on the staff, the number of referrals from these programs will also be limited. It might be interesting to note that the potential for patient referral for audiology and/or speech pathology services within VA medical centers is significant.

The VA Department of Medicine and Surgery conducts a nationwide census one day each year to determine specific items of patient information. Accompanying the request for patient information is a major question or issue for which additional information is gathered. Recently, as part of the annual census, the major question concerned the incidence of speech disorders among the veterans who were in the VA system on that day. Over 93,000 veterans were included in this census and the prevalence, type, and severity of speech disorders were ascertained. The questionnaire was completed by speech pathologists, wherever possible, but there were a considerable number of questionnaires completed by physicians, nurses and other medical center staff. The results of the census disclosed that approximately 25 percent, or 22,900, of the veterans in the VA system on that day exhibited a speech impairment that required the assistance of a speech pathologist. However, it was also reported that only about 3,000 of these veterans had either been seen, were being seen, or were in the process of being referred for speech pathology services.

In a similar manner, there have been a number of attempts to initiate hearing screening programs for veterans being admitted to medical centers. Almost all of the screening efforts have been discontinued because of the large numbers of hearing impairments that were discovered. The average failure rate reported, even after the possible effect of presbycusis was taken into consideration, was between 65 and 75 percent. Both the census data and the hearing screening data indicate the urgent need for audiology and speech-pathology services within the VA. The major reason for discontinuing the hearing screening programs was the fact that it was difficult to explain to a veteran that he had a hearing impairment that needed assistance but that, because of the lack of staff and other resources, nothing could be done to provide assistance. An awareness of the number of veterans needing professional services for their speech, language and/or hearing impairments is being made available to the appropriate individuals who are responsible for funding clinical programs nationwide. The number of audiology and speech pathology programs within the VA is growing rapidly because of the known urgent needs of the veterans. Additionally, program growth within the VA can also be attributed to the fact that the staff at the local medical centers has become aware of the communicative needs of the veteran patients.

VA audiology programs will receive about 60 percent of their referrals from the outpatient service and the remainder will be from the inpatient services within the medical center. Speech pathology receives 75 percent of their referrals from inpatient services within the medical center and the remainder from the outpatient service. For both audiology and speech pathology, the inpatients referred will usually need more sophisticated procedures, while the veterans seen as outpatients will be given the more routine audiology and/or speech pathology evaluations or treatment. The exception to these characteristics would be the veteran's need for a hearing aid evaluation or a compensation examination in the audiology program.

The difference between the outpatient and inpatient mix for audiology and speech pathology can be readily explained. The Veterans Administration is one of the few health care providers in the world that reimburses patients for coming to the medical centers for their treatment. Funds needed for beneficiary travel are extremely great and there is a concerted effort within the medical centers to minimize the number of outpatient visits that any one veteran might need. Because of this fact, speech pathology patients who may need long-term care are carefully monitored by the medical center and many of these patients are eventually referred to existing community programs rather than brought into the medical center. Aphasic patients in the medical center are discharged when it is thought medically advisable, and although there might be a need for continued speech pathology services, there is a limitation placed upon the number of times that the veteran can be seen on a long-term basis.

The types of patients seen by audiologists and speech pathologists within the VA system are not unlike the types of adult patients that are seen in the private sector. Approximately 60 percent of the patients seen in speech pathology are aphasic, with the remainder exhibiting organic speech involvements of many types. The majority of patient referrals for audiological examinations are sent for the more routine types of evaluations, and it is the responsibility of the audiologist to determine what specific audiological procedures should be conducted to ensure quality care.

In some instances, mainly in providing audiological services, there may be a restriction based upon the veteran's eligibility for such items as the issuance of a hearing aid. Entitlement for patient care provided by the medical center has been defined by congressional legislation and both the speech pathologist and the audiologist must be aware of these eligibility limitations when attempting to provide their speech, language and/or hearing services.

ADMINISTRATIVE RESPONSIBILITIES INVOLVED
IN THE MEDICAL CENTER SETTING

Many of the administrative responsibilities of the chief of the audiology and speech pathology service must function within the framework of the local medical center. The acquisition of the basic resources involving space, staff and equipment for the service must be channeled through an appropriate committee for consideration and ultimate approval. The audiology and speech pathology service is an entity of the medical center and it is the duty of the chief to portray the needs of the service with enough enthusiasm as to make resource recommendations attainable.

Personnel Selection

The selection of personnel for a VA audiology and speech pathology program follows the guidelines established for all federal agencies. It is the responsibility of the chief of the program to determine the need for additional staff or to initiate actions to employ personnel for existing vacancies. The need for additional professional and even clerical staff must be justified on existing workload and backlog of requests. In many instances, the chief can also solicit additional justification from other medical center service chiefs to amplify the need for an increase in audiology and/or speech pathology services through increased staffing.

Each medical center will have a committee that controls the number of positions each service is allowed. These position "ceilings" include part-time as well as full-time positions and each service must adhere to the recommendations of the manpower committee. Clerical vacancies are usually filled from within the medical center or the immediate community. When a professional vacancy exists within the audiology and speech pathology program, the chief, working closely with the medical center personnel service, sends a teletype to all VA facilities announcing the vacancy. It is standard VA procedure to allow audiologists and speech pathologists within the agency the first opportunity to apply for existing VA vacancies. If no suitable candidates for the vacant position can be found within the agency, the chief will request a list of candidates from the Office of Personnel Management (OPM) register through the medical center's personnel service. The request for register candidates must include the type and level of the vacant position. If the first set of candidate applications received from OPM are not satisfactory, additional applications are requested until a suitable candidate is found. It should be noted that there must be documentation forwarded to OPM outlining why a candidate is not considered suitable for the position. This documentation is made by the chief of the program and must be upheld by the medical center personnel service.

As can be seen, the chief of the program has the direct responsibility of selecting the staff of the service. The responsibility of the chief to each staff member is not restricted to just employment procedures. The chief must annually review the position description of each person in the service and make changes to reflect any new duties that may have been assigned, make recommendations for possible promotions or performance awards, recommend and implement continuing education experiences needed, and even initiate discharge procedures, if necessary. The quality of the professional and clerical staff within the audiology and speech pathology program is definitely one of the primary responsibilities of the chief.

Development and Acquisition of Needed Resources

The procedures involved in how the local medical centers receive their annual budgets will not be discussed in detail, but it is important for the medical center service chiefs to realize the overall budgeting cycle within the agency. In February each medical center will receive its budget for the fiscal year that begins the following October 1st. This allows the medical center programs to plan for the coming year. Audiology and speech pathology, for example, will know in February or March the number of training stipend awards for the coming year, and will therefore have adequate time to select the appropriate individuals for these positions. However, at the same time that the medical center is receiving its next fiscal year's budget, a budget proposal for the fiscal year beyond that funded must be submitted by the medical center for approval. In other words, a medical center will receive its fiscal year 1985 budget in February, 1985 and must at the same time submit its request for the fiscal year 1986 budget. Each medical center is therefore working with budget proposals for two years in the future. The service chiefs must realize this fact in their program planning. Some funds are available within each fiscal year to assist in employing staff and purchasing equipment. However, for the more significant expansions of staff or the purchasing of a large amounts of equipment, these must be planned over a possible two-year span.

Funds for supplies and other nonexpendables within the service are the most flexible resource available to the chief. Each year, after the budget has been sent to the medical center, an allotment of funds is provided each service for their needed supplies. Supply funds are controlled directly by the service chief and are fairly easily increased, within reason, by direct contact with the fiscal service.

Funds for staff, equipment, travel and specific continuing education expenses are controlled through specific medical center committees. If funding is desired in any of these categories, it is the responsibility of the service chief to justify the need to the appropriate committee. Obtaining funding in these areas is probably the greatest challenge that confronts a service chief in the administrative role. For example, if travel funds for the entire medical center are limited, it will be a challenge for the service chief to ensure that his staff receives an equitable share of what is available. The chief must be able to impart the importance of a staff member being funded for travel to the appropriate committee.

Management Briefings

In the majority of VA medical centers, a system of program management briefings is conducted. These briefings are an excellent vehicle for the service chief to use to alert the medical center administration about accomplishments and problems of their programs. Most medical centers will have two briefings per year for each program. The first briefing will allow the service chief to discuss problems anticipated in the future and to provide management a listing of the short- and long-range goals that are planned for the program. The short-range plans are usually confined to the current fiscal year, while the long-range plans could encompass a two-year period or more. The first briefing is held during the beginning of the fiscal year, with updated short- and long-range goals being presented at that time. During this first briefing, any problems that can be anticipated in the coming year or in the more distant future are also discussed. The second briefing is usually held midway in the fiscal year and, at that time, the progress that has been achieved for the original short-range goals are reviewed by management.

Participation in the briefing process is one of the greatest opportunities the service chiefs have for sharing their problems with the decision-making officials in the medical center. All of the medical center administrative officials are usually present during the briefings, and this creates the likelihood that the service chief will receive unified support for program needs. It is important for the service chiefs to realize that this is also an excellent opportunity to discuss the major accomplishments achieved by the program since the last briefing session. Modesty should not be exercised in these briefings. It is entirely possible that these same decision makers will be sitting on the committees that will be distributing resources during the coming fiscal year. The more appeal that a particular service has within the medical center, the greater the resource funding that may be directed to the program.

Decision-Making Process

Although the service chief is given the responsibility for making program decisions, it would be questionable if these decisions were made without input from the service staff. Periodic staff meetings must be held and it is usually recommended that these be scheduled weekly. During these meetings, the staff should be kept informed of what is happening within the medical center and, in some instances, what is happening throughout the VA. Service chiefs are encouraged to use these meetings as a chance to involve the staff in solving both administrative and clinical problems. All major decision making should be a result of staff input, or staff morale will become an additional problem.

Interprofessional Relationships

It has been mentioned previously that the organizational placement of audiology and speech pathology under the chief of staff allows the service chief the flexibility to work directly with the other service chiefs in the medical center. While VA audiologists and/or speech pathologists are considered professionals within the medical center, it is essential that interprofessional relationships be established and maintained that will provide continuing support for the audiology and speech pathology program. Each staff audiologist or speech pathologist must be encouraged to become involved with staff members in other services. In addition, it will be beneficial to the service if staff members show an interest in the medical center as a whole and become participants in committee assignments. The audiology and speech pathology program provides services on a referral basis and it is obvious that these referrals will be enhanced with good interprofessional relationships.

SUGGESTIONS TO FUTURE SPEECH-LANGUAGE-HEARING ADMINISTRATORS IN A MEDICAL SETTING

My suggestions to those who would like to administrate audiology and speech pathology programs can be summarized in two rather well-known sayings. The first is that "administrators are born, not made," and the second is that "a good administrator is at the right place, at the right time, doing the right thing."

I am a firm believer in the idea that administrators are born and not made. I have seen too many people who have enthusiastically enrolled in courses involving time management, labor relations, supervisory skills, etc., and at the end are still not good administrators or managers. There is a spark of something in a potentially good administrator that might have to be nurtured, but that spark is nevertheless present. The good administrator is an individual who is able to work easily with all types of people, and the belief that one is always working *with* others and not *for* them is important. This is particularly true when working with superiors. The good administrator knows that his or her talents can contribute to the mission of the medical center, but those talents may never be visible if the administrator is inhibited by the thought of working *for* someone. The same applies to the administrator's role with staff, whether they are professional audiologists and speech pathologists, clerks, secretaries, or even the housekeeping personnel assigned to his or her area. The administrator is working *with* them and vice versa.

The good administrator must be able to work on several tasks almost at the same time, and be able to complete each assignment well. I have never met a good manager who was ever completely out of something to do. A good manager must be able to do several things simultaneously, and at the same time establish flexible priorities on all tasks that are pending. I say flexible because there will be many times when circumstances change the relative importance of what needs to be done. This should be accepted as a fact of life and adapted to.

A good administrator loves challenges and loves what he or she is doing. The majority of good managers I have known would almost rather be working than going on vacation—but only 'almost'! Good managers are not clock watchers, because they love their work. I also believe that good administrators are not overly concerned with the amount of money they make, and though this will raise a few eyebrows I firmly believe it to be true. When the administrator begins a career, there will naturally be a concern about salary; however, when the joy of administration is experienced, money ceases to be the major reason for doing the job. If you really enjoy administration, the chances are that you are on the way toward achieving excellence in your work. If you are achieving excellence, you will eventually be rewarded. Part of that reward is often a salary adjustment.

As for the second saying, the good administrator must be prepared to be the person who is in the right place, at the right time, doing the right thing. The best way is to develop short- and long-range goals for yourself and your program on a continual basis. It is not enough to develop these goals once a year or once a month. Short- and long-range goals must be continually developed and changed. If you can master this continual development of short- and long-range goals, you will be ready to seize new opportunities as they arise. For example, suppose that you are running a program in which you perceive a clear need for computers. You establish this as a possible long-range goal, computers in your program for both the staff and patients to use. One day you learn that a company has just developed software to conduct hearing screening, and the total package of hardware and software is being marketed as a screening audiometer. You immediately go to your medical center and ask that patient care equipment, a screening audiometer, be purchased. It is more likely that you will receive patient care equipment than a computer. Now your long-range goal has become a short-range goal which you can probably achieve. If you do obtain a computer in this manner, you will have shown that you were in the right place, at the right time, doing the right thing. Good planning is the basis of good administration.

One last comment must be made about being a good administrator. It is important that you develop, among your other talents, the ability to listen. When you go into meetings, develop the ability to listen to other people to determine not only what they are saying but why they are saying it. Never be in a hurry to make declaratory statements unless there is no way to avoid it. When asked to make an immediate decision, be certain that you know and understand all of the possible alternatives. At the same time, be willing to compromise. It is better to get one-third of what you want in each of three meetings than to ask for all or nothing during the first meeting. Above all, you must also remember that you are a member of the medical center team. There will be times when you will have to subordinate your needs for the betterment of the medical center. This will happen and, when it does, the chances are great that eventually you will reap returns by showing you are a "team player."

REFERENCES

ANDERMAN, BERNARD. (1970). "The Veterans Administration audiology program," in *Hearing and Deafness*, eds. Hallowell Davis and S. R. Silverman. New York: Holt, Rinehart and Winston, 449–456.

CAUSEY, G. DONALD. (1976). "The hearing aid program of the Veterans Administration: Twenty years of service," *Bulletin of Prosthetics Research (BPR 10-25)*. Washington, D.C.: Veterans Administration, Department of Medicine and Surgery, 12–128.

COSTS TO OPERATE THE VETERANS ADMINISTRATION HEARING AID PROGRAM: *Report of the comptroller general of the United States (MWD-76-52). Washington,* D.C.: Veterans Administration. 1975.

NEWBY, HAYES. (1979). "Veterans Administration," in *Hearing and Hearing Impairment*, eds. Larry J. Bradford and William G. Hardy. New York: Grune and Stratton, 621–629.

WINTERCORN, E. S., AND L. B. BECK, eds. (1984). *Handbook of hearing aid measurement (IB 11-52)*. Washington, D.C.: Veterans Administration, Department of Medicine and Surgery.

10 Research and Training Programs of the National Institute of Neurological and Communicative Disorders and Stroke

Raymond R. Summers*

The National Institute of Neurological Diseases and Blindness was established by P.L. 81-692 in August 1950. The mission of the institute, known since 1975 as the National Institute of Neurological and Communicative Disorders and Stroke (NINCDS), is to conduct the support research and research training on the causes, prevention, diagnosis, and treatment of neurological and communicative disorders and stroke.

In carrying out its mission, the institute is involved in a number of specific activities: (1) It awards grants to support extramural research projects, program projects, and specialized research centers; (2) it awards training grants to institutions and fellowships to individuals to increase academic and research manpower; (3) it supports seminars and workshops designed to coordinate, exchange, and disseminate information when such activities are directed toward objectives which are clearly within the mission of the institute; (4) it enters into contracts to support research which NINCDS program personnel identify as being important in achieving their mission; (5) it conducts intramural research in nine basic science laboratories and seven clinical units at the National Institutes of Health; and (6) it collects and disseminates research information in the neurological and communicative basic and clinical sciences. Of these six activities, this chapter deals only with the first three,

*Dr. Summers is chief, Scientific Review Branch, National Institute of Neurological and Communicative Disorders and Stroke, Bethesda, Maryland.

the procedures for obtaining support for extramural research, training, and seminars and workshops. The NINCDS commits approximately 75 percent of its annual appropriation to supporting extramural research and training activities, and investigators and training program directors may apply for available funds to support their research projects and/or training programs. Grants and contracts can be awarded to both nonprofit and for-profit applicants.

To carry out its mission, the NINCDS receives an annual appropriation which is a line item in the budget for the Department of Health and Human Services (DHHS) for the fiscal year October 1 through the following September 30. As a line item, the amount appropriated by the Congress cannot be increased or decreased by personnel in either the DHHS or the National Institutes of Health (NIH). When Congress fails to enact appropriate legislation by the beginning of the fiscal year, it passes a "continuing resolution" which enables the institute to continue to operate at a specified budget level, for example, the level of the previous year's budget, the level of the budget submitted by the president, or the level of the budget approved by either the House of Representatives or the Senate. The lack of an appropriation usually does not create a problem but rather an inconvenience. In the past ten fiscal years, beginning with FY 1976, the department received only six appropriations, thus operating under a continuing resolution for four years.

In addition to providing an appropriation or passing a continuing resolution, Congress sometimes takes other actions that affect the way the institute carries out its mission. For instance, Congress might request that specific studies be carried out or that specified amounts of the institute's appropriation be used for awards in a specific disease area or to study a specific technological development. The institute must sometimes deal with ceilings placed on the total number of awards that can be made or with personnel ceilings or employment freezes.

The NINCDS supports a number of specific research and training activities. All grant applications are initiated by a principal investigator (research), a program director (training, program project, or workshop), or an individual interested in postdoctoral training (fellowship). The following are the types of activities supported:

Research Activities

Research Project Grant—Supports a discrete, circumscribed research project performed by a principal investigator in an area of his or her specific interest and competency.

Conference Grant—Supports national or international symposia, conferences, and workshops.

First Independent Research Support and Transition (FIRST) Award—Provides a sufficient period of support for newly independent investigators to develop their research capabilities and demonstrate the merit of their research ideas.

Small Business Innovation Research Grant (Phase I)—Supports projects, limited in time and amount, to establish the technical merit and feasibility of ideas which may ultimately lead to commercial products or services.

Small Business Innovation Research Grant (Phase II)—Supports in-depth development of ideas whose feasibility has been established during Phase I awards and which are likely to result in commercial products or services.

Research Program Project Grant—Supports a research program in which a multidisciplinary team of experienced investigators works collaboratively in a clearly defined area of mutual scientific interest. In a program project, achievement of the objective of the research effort is facilitated by sharing ideas, data, and specialized core resources such as equipment, laboratories, clinical facilities, and administrative services. An essential requirement is a central theme toward which the total scientific effort is directed.

Specialized Center Grant—Supports all or part of a full range of research and development activities from very basic to clinical; may involve ancillary supportive activities such as patient care necessary to the primary research effort. The spectrum of activities comprises a multidisciplinary attack on a specific disease or biomedical problem. These grants differ from program project grants in that they are usually developed in response to an announcement of a programmatic need of the institute and subsequently they receive continuous attention from the staff.

Training Activities

Institutional National Research Service Award—Enables grantee institutions to award to individuals, selected by the program director, fellowship support for postdoctoral research training in specified disciplines. A limited number of predoctoral stipends may be provided. Also supports short-term training of medical, dental, and veterinary students during periods when they are not involved in their professional preparation.

Postdoctoral Individual National Research Service Award—Provides postdoctoral research training to individuals to broaden their scientific background and extend their potential for research in health-related areas.

Research Career Development Award—Fosters the development of scientists qualified either to pursue independent research which would extend the research program of the sponsoring institution, or to direct an essential part of that research program.

Clinical Investigator Development Award—Prepares clinically trained persons for research and teaching careers in areas of medical science related to the neurological and communicative disorders. This award, made to an institition, provides a superior candidate with an opportunity for up to five years of special study and supervised experience tailored to individual needs. Candidates for this award are usually clinicians who have M.D. degrees. However, in the communicative sciences, clinicians who have attained the Ph.D. degree are eligible to apply for an award.

To understand fully the NIH procedures for obtaining grant support, one should be familiar with the structure of the Extramural Activities Program of an institute and be familiar with the responsibilities of the component parts. The NINCDS is typical of the institutes in its structure. The Extramural Activities Program consists of four branches that support five program areas. The four branches are the Administrative Services Branch, Contracts Management Branch, Grants Management Branch, and Scientific Review Branch. The five program areas are the

Communicative Disorders Program; Convulsive, Developmental, and Neuromuscular Disorders Program; Demyelinating, Atrophic, and Dementing Disorders Program; Fundamental Neurosciences Program; and Stroke and Trauma Program.

Each of the five programs has a specific mission and all applications assigned to the institute are also assigned to a program. The mission of the Communicative Disorders Program (CDP) is to support research and research training on the causes, prevention, diagnosis, and treatment of disorders in those systems by which humans communicate with each other or interact with their environment. All research and training applications that are related to this mission are assigned to the Communicative Disorders Program. The program has an external seven-member advisory committee which reviews its mission and long-range objectives. If, in conjunction with its advisory committee, it seems desirable to the public to solicit applications in a specific research area, the institute can issue a program announcement or a "request for applications." Personnel also accomplish the program's mission by discussing research initiatives with investigators attending professional meetings, by encouraging the submission of an application from an investigator known to be engaged in an important area of research, or by responding to letters or telephone inquiries about research interests. All program announcements and requests for applications are printed in the publication, "NIH Guide to Grants and Contracts." The CDP administers approximately 360 grants and contracts in the following categories:

Disturbances of balance, including postural vertigo and Menière's disease

Ear, nose, and throat diseases, including cancer of the head and neck, laryngeal papillomas, temporal bone pathology, and tumors of the outer, middle, and inner ear

Hearing disorders, including presbycusis, otosclerosis, and impairment caused by otitis media

Speech disorders such as dysarthria and speech abnormalities caused by laryngeal disease

Rhythm disorders such as stuttering

Language disorders, including aphasia resulting from stroke and delayed language development

Disorders of taste, and smell, varying from distortions of these senses to total loss

NINCDS-supported scientists are also studying control of balance in both humans and animals, electrical activitity in the auditory system during hearing, brain activity while a subject speaks or listens to speech, the biochemistry of the auditory system, the histochemistry of taste and smell, auditory or cochlear implants, and tactile aids for the hearing-impaired.

All research and training grant applications related to the mission of the Communicative Disorders Program are assigned to that program. In addition, each application is further assigned to a health scientist administrator in that program and it becomes a part of the portfolio of applications which that individual administers. That person, whether a speech/language pathologist, audiologist, otolaryngologist, or sensory physiologist, is the individual whom program directors or principal investigators contact if they have questions about either their grant, NIH or NINCDS policy, or subsequent application procedures. They are the individuals who review progress reports and who interact with grants management specialists if there are fiscal questions about a grant or the activities being supported.

The mission of the Communicative Disorders Program is so comprehensive that practically all applications involving any phase of the communication process are assigned to the NINCDS. A small number of research applications involving language or communication might be assigned to other institutes. For instance, applications involving the development of language or the acquisition of speech might be assigned to the National Institute of Child Health and Human Development. Applications dealing with geriatric or aging disabilities that affect speech or communication might be assigned to the National Institute of Aging.

At a recent meeting of the National Advisory Council, action was taken on 102 applications which were assigned to the Communicative Disorders Program. Of these applications, two were for supplemental funds, three for program projects, one for a conference grant, and 22 for the support of research in the chemosenses. The remaining 74 applicants were for the support of investigator-initiated research in the communicative sciences. Such research is extremely complex as evidenced by the wide variation in the professional preparation of the principal investigators. Of the 74 applicants, 15 (20 percent) investigators were trained in speech pathology, audiology, or linguistics; 23 (31 percent) investigators were trained in some aspect of psychology; 16 (22 percent) were trained in the basic sciences (anatomy, chemistry, physiology); 11 (15 percent) in some area of engineering; 8 (11 percent) in some area of medicine; and 1 (1 percent) in a social science. Of these 74 applications, 67 were recommended for approval and 34 (51 percent) were funded.

Seeking NINCDS support for a research or training activity requires that an application be submitted. The application goes through a peer review process and an award is made if the application has high technical merit and high program relevance. The following is a brief description of the characteristics of these three procedures, application, review, and award.

SUBMITTING APPLICATIONS

Specific application forms are necessary for applying for NINCDS support and it is essential that proper forms be used for the specific type of grant being sought, that is, research or training.

The most commonly used form is PHS 398, DHHS/PHS Grant Application, the form used for seeking support for an investigator-initiated research project. This form is also used in applying for support for other activities and, therefore, the basic instructions for completing the form may include additional policies and instructions depending upon the specific activity for which support is being sought. All instructions for completing the form should be followed. Forms for seeking National Research Service Award support are PHS 416 and PHS 6025 for individual postdoctoral fellowship suport and institutional training grant support respectively.

The NIH has a unit, the Division of Research Grants (DRG), which is best described as a "support" unit for all bureaus, institutes and divisions of NIH. Although grant application forms can usually be obtained from an institution's grants and contracts office, if they are not available there they can be obtained from the DRG. All applications are sent to the DRG where they are assigned to an initial review group (IRG) for evaluation, and to an awarding organization, for example, a component that has ultimate responsibility for making an award. Applications in the communicative sciences would normally be assigned to one of three standing committees for their initial review: the Hearing Research Study Section (HAR), the Sensory Disorders and Language Study Section (CMS), or the Communicative Disorders Review Committee (CDRC). The Hearing Research Study Section and the Sensory Disorders and Language Study Section are in the Division of Research Grants, whereas the Communicative Disorders Review Committee is one of three standing committees in the NINCDS. The HAR and CMS study sections review applications for regular research grants and Research Career Development awards. The CDRC reviews applications for program projects, specialized centers, conferences and workshops, National Research Service Award training grants, and Clinical Investigator Development awards. Applications for National Research Service Award postdoctoral fellowships are generally reviewed by "flexible" study sections in the Division of Research Grants. Such study sections consist of up to fifty members and are subdivided into four or five subcommittees organized according to specific areas of training. Thus all individuals seeking training in some phase of communication would have their applications evaluated by the same scientific review committee.

INITIAL REVIEW OF APPLICATIONS

Once applications are assigned to an initial review group, either a study section or an institute review committee, they are the responsibility of the executive secretary who handles the review body. The responsibilities of an executive secretary are well defined and structured, the primary responsibility being to ensure that each application receives an appropriate and fair scientific review. However, the structured nature of this position does not imply that it is rigid and unchanging. Recent congressional and presidential directives, such as the Freedom of Information Act, the Privacy Act, and the Government in the Sunshine Act, as well as policy changes related to the involvement of human subjects in research, animal welfare, and biohazards, have had a significant impact upon the review process. In addition, the automatic release of summary statements with priority scores and percentile rankings to the principal investigator as soon as they are prepared places a substantial responsibility on the executive secretary for ensuring that the review process and the summary statement are of exceptionally high quality.

The evaluation of grant applications, sometimes referred to as peer review, is based on dual review—two sequential levels of review. Because of the magnitude, diversity, and complexity of its research mission as well as its pursuit of excellence, the first level of review involves a national group of scientists, usually nonfederal, actively engaged in research and established in panels according to scientific disciplines or research areas for the purpose of evaluating the scientific and technical merit of applications. These panels are legislatively mandated and are generally referred to as scientific review groups or initial review groups. In the Division of Research Grants, they are identified as *study sections*. Currently DRG has sixty-six chartered study sections some of which have one or more subcommittees resulting in eighty-seven chartered review groups.

The study section or scientific review group usually has the expertise among its members to evaluate all applications it is responsible for reviewing. Where such expertise is missing, the executive secretary might invite ad hoc reviewer(s) with expertise in that area to join the review group, or the executive secretary might solicit written comments from experts in the area and make these comments available to the scientific review committee. The evaluation of applications is accomplished independently of personnel in the Communicative Disorders Program who may have been instrumental in stimulating the application. One of the basic policies governing NIH operating procedures is that review responsibilities are organizationally separate, that program personnel are not allowed to exert an influence on the scientific review of applications and review personnel are not to influence the programming process. The individual who stimulates an application or who might be involved in the administration of a program if the application is funded cannot make any statements or be involved in any procedure that might influence the scientific review of the application.

The scientific review of most applications in the communicative sciences is by one of the three committees earlier identified, and the membership of these committees ordinarily ranges from sixteen to twenty members. The primary requirement for serving on an initial review group is competence as an independent investigator in a scientific or clinical discipline or research specialty. Assessment of such competence is based on the quality of research accomplished, publications in refereed journals, and other significant activities and achievements. Such individuals have usually obtained a doctorate. Members must have mature judgment, balanced perspective, objectivity, ability to work effectively in a group context, commitment to complete work assignments, assurance that the confidentiality of applications will be protected, and no real or potential conflicts of interest.

Members of initial review groups are selected by the executive secretary who is the federal official in charge of study section or technical merit review committee meetings, as required under the Federal Advisory Committee Act. The chairperson for a study section or an initial review group is selected by the executive secretary with the concurrence of his or her supervisor. The chairperson must have had previous experience with review groups or similar bodies. The individual should be highly respected by members of the scientific community and by members of the review group and should be a leader in the field. Chairpersons are usually appointed for the last two years of their four-year term.

All initial review group members serve a four-year term on a rotating basis and they may be reappointed to the same or to a different committee after a lapse of one year between appointments. In their evaluation of applications, committees consider such factors as: the scientific, technical, medical significance, and originality of the proposed research; the appropriateness and adequacy of the research protocol and methodology; the qualifications and experience of the principal investigator and staff in the area of the proposed research; the reasonableness of the proposed budget and duration of requested support; and, where an application involves activities that could have an adverse effect upon humans, animals, or the environment, the adequacy of the proposed means for protecting against or minimizing such effects.

The National Institutes of Health has a continually updated NIH consultant file which contains the names and résumés of potential reviewers or study section members. This file, through a comprehensive coding system, identifies each potential consultant's areas of research expertise. The file identifies approximately 550 specific research areas. This consultant file is maintained by a contractor who can provide two types of information to executive secretaries, a list of potential reviewers by speciality area and a curriculum vitae for anyone whose name appears in the file. For individuals who desire to be included in the file, the contractor provides a nomination form. All requests for these nomination forms should be sent to the National Institutes of Health, from where they will be forwarded to the contractor.

In carrying out scientific review responsibilities, project site visits are sometimes required. This is especially true of applications for program projects and specialized centers because applications to support such programs are complex and costly. Site visit teams include both IRG committee members and ad hoc consultants. The number of site visitors is that required to assess all technical aspects of the application. In the instance of a regular research grant application, this may involve two or three site visitors, but in the case of a program project or a specialized center, this could involve ten to fifteen site visitors.

Site visits require considerable time and attention on the part of the program director and all associates involved in the program. The program director has every right to expect that the visit will have a definite purpose and that its results will have a considerable, if not deciding, influence on the final disposition of the application.

Site visit teams evaluate, through discussions with the program director and all associates or collaborators, their knowledge of the field, experience, and their exact responsibilities for the program. During the site visit, each investigator is queried about concerns reviewers have regarding the research protocol. The visitors assess the research facilities and laboratories, paying particular attention to the availability of essential equipment for conducting the research; observe research techniques and procedures that are vital to the success of the research; make determinations about the appropriateness of the budgets; and assess the length of time for which support is being requested.

A site visit is a friendly fact-finding mission, not an adversary proceeding, an inquisition, or a bargaining session. Following the visit, a site visit report is prepared which conveys the visitors' recommendations to an initial review committee.

The Privacy Act of 1974 provides certain safeguards for individuals against invasions of personal privacy. These safeguards include (1) the right of individuals to determine what information about them is maintained in federal agencies' files and to known how that information is used; and (2) the right of individuals to have access to such records and to correct, amend, or request deletion of information in their records that is inaccurate, irrelevant, or outdated. Site visit reports are among the documents that must be made available under the Privacy Act. Site visit reports are, therefore, sent to applicants if they are requested. The site visit report, however, is considered only a "working" document and once its usefulness to the initial review group has been fulfilled, it is destroyed. The site visitors' comments and recommendations, as reflected in the site visit report, are superseded by the initial review group's evaluation as reflected in the summary statement.

Members of an initial review committee can make one of three recommendations. Applications can be recommended for approval, disapproval, or deferral. All applications recommended for approval are assumed to have sufficient merit to be worthy of support. A vote for approval is equivalent to a recommendation that a grant be awarded provided sufficient funds are available. The recommendation can be for the time and amount requested or for an adjusted time and amount.

All applications recommended for approval include a recommendation about the budget and about the duration of support. Reviewers determine whether the requested budget is realistic and appropriate for the conduct of the research. They may recommend that certain personnel be deleted from the budget if they do not appear necessary to perform the research, or that the amount of effort by certain personnel be reduced if it is judged that the requested effort is excessive for the needs of the project. Such a recommendation is made even if no salary is requested.

If reviewers recommend reductions in the amount of the support requested or the length of time required for the research, they must provide specific reasons for the modifications and these will be documented in the summary statement. Reductions may be recommended (1) when reviewers recommend deleting parts of a project; (2) when the funds requested in any budget category are not justified by the research described in the application; (3) when the principal investigator has provided insufficient information in the application about the work to be done in future years; (4) when reviewers think the research can be completed in fewer years than requested; and (5) when the principal investigator is entering a new research area and, because of questions regarding the feasibility of the projects, the reviewers would like to review the preliminary work. It is rare that a project is recommended for less than three years, because the length of the review cycle would mandate that the investigator would have to begin the preparation of a renewal application almost immediately to receive continuous funding.

Following a recommendation of approval of an application, each member of the scientific review group assigns the application a priority. Each member rates each application privately. The scale utilized is from 1.0 (most meritorious) to 5.0 (least meritorious) with increments of 0.1. If the vote for approval is not unanimous, reviewers who did not vote approval must record a priority rating which may be, but need not be, 5.0. Reviewers abstaining from voting do not record a priority. In assigning priorities, the priority is given to the project as recommended by the review group rather than to the application as originally submitted. Reviewers should (1) assign priorities based strictly on thoughtful and objective considerations of the review criteria, not on emotional or institute budgetary considerations; (2) judge the merit of each application independently from other proposals and according to their own standards of quality; and (3) rate privately and not discuss their specific priorities with other reviewers. Applications are not compared with each other, they are judged on the basis of their own merits.

After the meeting of the scientific review committee, the individual reviewers' ratings for each application are averaged and multiplied by 100, which results in a three-digit priority. Following the computation of the priority, the percentile ranking of each approved research grant application is determined. The priority and the percentile are included on the summary statement which is forwarded to the investigator as soon as it is prepared. The summary statement is also made available to the Advisory Council for its recommendation. The priority and the percentile are important indicators of the quality of the application and guide the council and institute in their decisions regarding the order in which applications are funded.

The assignment of a percentile ranking is the last step in the process of evaluating applications for scientific merit, and all aspects of the initial review can have an influence on the reliability and validity of the resulting ranking. The priority score system alone has, at times, been criticized, particularly for perceived inconsistencies in the initial review group's rating behavior. These concerns have led the NINCDS and some other institutes at NIH to use the percentile ranking of research applications as the measure of scientific merit. Training grant applications continue to be funded on the basis of the assigned priority score.

Applications that lack sufficient merit to be worthy of support are recommended for disapproval. Disapproval may also be recommended when gravely hazardous or unethical procedures are involved, or when no funds can be recommended, such as in the case of a supplemental application where the work is deemed to be unnecessary. If the initial review committee determines that the named principal investigator will not be clearly responsible for the scientific and technical direction of the project, the application would be recommended for disapproval on that basis. No priority is given to applications recommended for disapproval.

If the initial review committee cannot make a recommendation without obtaining additional information, the application is recommended for deferral. The information required to make a judgment may be obtained by telephone, by a project site visit, by outside opinions, or by the submission of additional material. Deferred applications are usually reviewed again at the next meeting of the initial review committee.

If an investigator has questions about the technical merit review of his or her application, there are two options. The matter can be discussed with personnel in the Communicative Disorders Program or, if a site visit has been made and the investigator has concerns about some aspect of the visit, he or she can write a rebuttal letter to the initial review group if the application has not already been reviewed. In either of the above instances, if the investigator's concern is not satisfactorily resolved, a rebuttal letter can be sent to the council. Rebuttal letters are addressed to the health scientist administrator who has been assigned responsibility for that specific application. Rebuttal letters, if received in time, are mailed to all council members at the time summary statements are mailed. Rebuttal letters received too late to be mailed are made available to council members at the time of the council meeting.

Protection of human subjects.   In the communicative disorders, it is not unusual for research to involve human subjects, and the Department of Health and Human Services has regulations which provide a systematic means, based on established ethical principles, to safeguard the rights and welfare of individuals who participate as subjects in research activities. The Office for Protection from Research Risks, NIH, has departmentwide authority and responsibility for implementing regulations concerning human subjects. For purposes of NIH research, a *human subject* is a living individual about whom an investigator conducting research obtains data through intervention or direct interaction, or about whom an investigator obtains identifiable private information. This involves the use of human organs, tissues, and body fluids from individually identifiable human subjects as well as to graphic, written, or recorded information derived from individually identifiable human subjects. Also assessed by review groups are additional protections required for certain classes of human research involving fetuses, pregnant women, human *in vitro* fertilization, and prisoners.

Research activities normally involving little or no risk, in which the only involvement of human subjects will be one or more of the following categories, are exempt from the human subjects regulations:

1. Research conducted in established or commonly accepted educational settings and involving normal educational practices.
2. Research involving the use of education tests if the information is recorded in such a manner that subjects cannot be identified.
3. Research involving survey or interview procedures except where certain conditions exist.
4. Research involving the observation of public behavior except where certain conditions exist.

5. Research involving the collection or study of existing data, documents, records, pathological specimens, or diagnostic specimens, if these sources are publicly available.

Each institution engaged in research covered by regulations protecting human subjects shall provide a written assurance that it will comply with the requirements set forth in the regulations. For the most part, this is done through an Institutional Review Board (IRB), composed of at least five members with varying backgrounds who review applications for that institution. The certification of IRB review of declaration or exemption is conveyed to the institute and initial group by completing a "Protection of Human Subjects Assurance/Certification/Declaration" form, HHS 596, which must be submitted with all applications unless it is designated on the face page of the application that the institution has an exemption which applies to the research.

Animal welfare. It is the policy of the Public Health Service that the humane care and use of animals in research and training programs is the responsibility of the principal investigator and the grantee institution. The Office of Protection From Research Risks, NIH, has departmentwide authority and responsibility for implementing the regulations concerning animal care.

For NIH purposes, an *animal* is any live, vertebrate animal used or intended for use in research, experimentation, testing, training, or related purposes. No grant involving the use of animals will be made unless a responsible official of the applicant institution has provided an acceptable written assurance to the NIH that (1) the institution is committed to complying with the Animal Welfare Act (P.L. 89-544, as amended) and (2) the institution has appointed and will maintain a committee of five members, including at least one veterinarian, to provide oversight of its animal care program.

It is the responsibility of the executive secretary to code each application to identify whether the IRG noted any concerns or comments about human subjects or animal welfare. A "concern" is an IRG finding that requires resolution by the program staff before an award is made. A "comment" is an IRG observation that is communicated in the summary statement as a suggestion to the principal investigator or program director.

SECONDARY REVIEW OF APPLICATIONS

The second level of the dual review systems is carried out by a legislated advisory board or advisory council, that is, in the NINCDS, the National Advisory Neurological and Communicative Disorders and Stroke Council. This council consists of sixteen individuals, both scientific and lay representatives, who are noted for their expertise, interest, or activity in matters related to the mission of the institute. The council's recommendations are based not only on a consideration of the scientific merit of applications, as judged by the scientific review groups which assign priorities to all applications recommended for approval, but also on the relevance of the proposed research or training activity, outlined in the application, to the institute's programs and priorities. The dual review system separates the scientific assessment of proposed projects from policy decisions about scientific areas to be supported and the level of resources to be allocated, and it permits a more objective evaluation than would result from a single level of review. This system of review also provides responsible NINCDS officials with the best available advice about scientific as well as societal values and needs.

The ultimate objective of the Extramural Activities Program of the NINCDS is the funding of investigator-initiated research projects and training programs. What specific applications are supported through grants is determined in large measure by the research community's perception of the most promising scientific or training opportunities. This perception is expressed in the peer review process. This involves the initial review groups or study sections, which assign priority scores to all approved applications, and the National Advisory Council.

In any one fiscal year, 65 to 70 percent of the funds available to the institute are used to fund currently supported programs that have subsequent years of recommended support. The remaining 30 to 35 percent are available for the support of new and competing applications. At the council meeting some applications are designated as meriting special consideration for funding. Such applications are those having high scientific merit and high program relevance but which do not meet the funding cutoff. These are carefully selected applications, identified by the program staff and by the council, which fall above the percentile ranking cutoff for a given application cycle, but which deserve further consideration for funding, if funds are available. A variety of criteria are used for identifying applications for special consideration and the most important of these are the following:

1. Program balance and program needs. The Communicative Disorders Program attempts to maintain a general balance among its various areas of responsibility. Of special concern is the problem of maintaining a balance between clinical and basic research. Because clinical research may be technically more difficult to design and execute, clinical research applications tend to have poorer priorities than do those in basic research. One way of keeping the necessary clinical research in the portfolio is through the special consideration mechanism. Program personnel also identify other areas of special need, for example, where there are specific congressional or departmental initiatives, or where the project fills an unmet need in a research portfolio.

2. Funds already invested. In general, special consideration would be requested for continued support of an ongoing project, rather than for broadening and extending support to new projects when funds are not available to support both approaches.

3. Other research in the same area. Although no two research projects overlap completely, if the Communicative Disorders Program is already supporting several projects in a given area, it would generally not request special consideration for another one in the same area.

4. Assisting new investigators. First applications from promising new investigators may be singled out for special consideration as a mechanism for getting them started in the field.

The designation of an application for special consideration does not mean that it will necessarily be funded, since money is not available to fund all such applications. Communicative Disorders Program personnel, following each council meeting, recommend to the director, NINCDS, those applications to be funded. The staff makes all funding decisions and, although the staff values the council's advice, its advice cannot be followed strictly. The staff's funding decisions are reported to the council at its next meeting and the council can ask the staff to justify its decisions. The responsibility for making funding decisions cannot be delegated to an outside advisory group.

The institute's procedures for working with the council in the review of applications are based on NIH and NINCDS guidelines which have been developed to meet legal requirements, and to provide an appropriate input from the council in the funding process. By law, no applications may be funded unless the council has recommended their approval. Generally the council concurs with the initial review group or study section's recommendation for approval, and also with the priority and subsequent percentile ranking assigned to the application.

There are other methods for selecting applications to fund. Funding could be accomplished exclusively on the basis of technical merit, in which case applications would be funded according to the percentile ranking until available funds are obligated. The extreme would be to ignore the technical merit, that is, priority and percentile, entirely and fund those applications which have the greatest perceived program relevance. The NINCDS uses a combination of these extremes. Some applications are funded exclusively on the basis of their technical merit or percentile, which might be identified as the "automatic cutoff," and others on a combined basis of percentile and program relevance. The institute gives priority to funding the very best science regardless of discipline or program area. The actual percentile for the automatic cutoff varies from council to council and from year to year, depending on the availability of funds.

FISCAL MANAGEMENT OF GRANTS

The NIH expects the applicant institution to anticipate the full extent of its financial requirements when applying for a grant, to justify all costs in terms of essentiality to the project or program, and to budget for such costs in the application. The award of a grant constitutes prior approval for the expenditure of funds for costs which are included in the recommended budget. All applications to be funded receive an administrative and programmatic review by NINCDS personnel prior to an award being made. The administrative review, carried out by grants management specialists, involves such activities as making certain that all departmental policies are followed, for example, human subject certification is appropriate and all budget items are appropriate. The programmatic review, carried out by Communicative Disorders Program personnel, involves a determination, for example, of whether the application is part of the program's funding plan and whether the research overlaps with similar or identical research being funded by another federal agency.

The budget of a grant-supported activity includes all allowable direct costs incident to the performance of the research or training activity, plus the allocable portion of the allowable indirect costs of the applicant organization. All costs must be reasonable and necessary. Direct costs are any costs that can be specifically identified with a particular project or program and they include, but are not limited to, salaries, travel, equipment, and supplies directly benefiting the project or activity. Budgets for training grants also include categories for trainee expenses, that is, stipends, tuition and fees, and trainee travel. Indirect costs are those incurred by an organization for common or joint objectives which cannot be identified specifically with a particular project or program. Facilities, maintenance costs, depreciation, and administrative expenses are examples of costs that are usually treated as indirect costs.

Applicants who compete successfully for an award receive a "notice of grant award" which identifies the amount of the award, by budget category, for a specified budget period, usually one year, and the amount recommended annually for subsequent years of recommended support, usually two to four years. The initial budget period plus the additional years of recommended support are referred to as the competitive segment. The initial competitive segment and any extensions to it are referred to as the project period, a period identified on the award statement. The amounts awarded in each budget category are those deemed necessary and appropriate following the administrative and programmatic review of the amount required for a given budget period.

The activity to be pursued is that described in the application and recommended for approval with modifications which appear in the summary statement or as subsequently approved during a subsequent competitive segment. Once the notice of grant award is issued, the investigator or program director may desire to make post-award programmatic changes and to rebudget funds within and among budget categories to meet unanticipated requirements necessary to successfully carry out the research or training program. Such changes and rebudgeting must enhance the progress of the project toward meeting its stated objective. Advice on how to request the necessary prior approval and what constitutes appropriate documentation of it may be obtained from the grantee institution's office of sponsored programs or the equivalent unit. Whenever prior NINCDS approval is required, a written request must be submitted for institute review and appropriate action. The request must be signed by the principal investigator and also by an official authorized to sign for the grantee institution, and it must be received before actually initiating the programmatic change for rebudgeting the funds. These requests always receive an administrative and programmatic review. The grants management officer's signature must appear on any response approving or denying a business management activity.

Whenever grantees contemplate rebudgeting or other post-award changes and are uncertain about the allowability of types or costs of activities, they are encouraged to consult, in advance, the institute's grants management officer, one of the two individuals whose signatures appear on the bottom of the notice of grant award. This is particularly true when such actions or items are not specifically mentioned in the regulations, cost principles, or policy documents.

The staffs of the Communicative Disorders Program and the Extramural Activities Program are available to assist investigators and program directors in helping the institute carry out its mission in the communicative sciences, that of conducting and supporting research and research training on the causes, prevention, diagnosis, and treatment of communicative disorders.

Personnel in the Communicative Disorders Program are available to assist applicants in submitting the best possible applications, and they are available to make suggestions about how applications might be strengthened. Once applications are submitted, personnel in the Scientific Review Branch are responsible for assuring that applications receive the best possible scientific review. Personnel in the Grants Management Branch are responsible for assuring that no fiscal constraints restrict or interfere with the conduct of the research or research training activity that is funded.

11 American Speech-Language-Hearing Association and Its National Office

Frederick T. Spahr*

The American Speech-Language-Hearing Association was founded in 1925 as an organization named the American Academy of Speech Correction. The association's name was changed in 1927 to American Society for the Study of Disorders of Speech; in 1934, to American Speech Correction Association; in 1947, to the American Speech and Hearing Association; and, in 1978, the organization assumed its present name with the acronym ASHA.

In 1987, it is projected that the association will be comprised of over 53,000 audiologists, speech-language pathologists, and language, hearing, and speech scientists. A small percentage of ASHA members belongs to related professions such as psychology, medicine, and engineering, with these members having demonstrated a commitment to and/or interest in human communication and its disorders. In 1987, the association's budget is expected to approximate $9,450,000, and the staff size will exceed 100.

ASHA is established as a 501(c)(6) organization with two 501(c)(3) subsidiaries. The nonprofit tax status of these organizations is important because ASHA's tax status allows the organization to engage in lobbying efforts with Congress and state legislatures to effect laws and regulations benefitting professionals and those with communication disabilities. Likewise, the 501(c)(3) tax status for

*Dr. Spahr is the executive director of the American Speech-Language-Hearing Association, Rockville, Maryland.

the American Speech-Language Hearing Foundation (ASHF) and the National Association for Hearing and Speech Action (NAHSA) reflects their establishment as charitable trusts so that gifts to the foundation and NAHSA, whether in the form of direct contribution, property, or bequests, are fully tax deductible under Internal Revenue Service regulations. ASHF was founded in 1956 and is part of the formal structure of the American Speech-Language-Hearing Association as specified in Article XI of ASHA's bylaws. The foundation focuses primarily on professional development by fostering research, scholarship, and clinical achievement. NAHSA was founded in 1910 and is an older organization than either ASHA or the foundation. NAHSA existed independently until 1979 when ASHA formally assumed management of the then financially troubled organization. Since 1979, NAHSA's debtors have been paid and the organization is operating on a basis of revenues exceeding expenses. A board of directors, comprised primarily of individuals who are *not* speech-language pathologists and audiologists, functions independently of ASHA in regard to program, policy, and fiscal matters. Designated as ASHA's consumer affiliate, NAHSA is primarily concerned with increasing the visibility of communication disorders, heightening public awareness of the availability of professional diagnostic and remedial services, and advocating action which will improve the quality of life for those individuals with speech, language or hearing impairments.

Internationally, ASHA is a member of the International Association of Logopedics and Phoniatrics (IALP). ASHA is also a member of other international and national organizations concerned with disabilities as these relate to education, health, and rehabilitation. In addition, ASHA maintains close relationships with speech, language, and hearing organizations in other countries, and three members of ASHA's legislative council (policymaking body) are elected from countries outside the United States.

Speech-language-hearing associations exist in all fifty states. These state associations are independent of ASHA, although ASHA provides formal recognition of state associations who seek such on a voluntary basis. ASHA recognition largely rests on the basis of membership requirements for individual affiliation with the state organizations (i.e., the master's degree or equivalent for voting membership). Good working relationships between state associations and ASHA (as well as among state associations themselves) are critical to the continued vitality of the profession. These relationships are critical in certain areas such as (a) standards for providers of speech, language, and hearing services (ASHA certification, state licensure, state department of education certification); (b) for programs that provide services to the communicatively disabled such as Medicare (federal) and Medicaid (state); and (c) state-regulated health insurance. State and national relationships are fostered through such groups as the Council of State Association Presidents and the ASHA Committee on State-National Relationships.

ASHA has extensive liaison activity internal and external to the profession. There are a number of related professional organizations (RPOs) that have formed to focus on single issue concerns. These organizations are comprised primarily of professionals in speech, language, and hearing. ASHA also belongs to a number of coalitions that are comprised of associations having mutual interests related to special education, health, and/or rehabilitation. For example, ASHA is a member of the National Committee for Research in Neurological and Communicative Disorders (NCR). This organization is comprised of thirty voluntary associations and thirty professional associations with the single focus to increase federal appropriations for biomedical research related to human communication and its disorders, conducted through the auspices of the National Institute of Neurological and Communicative Disorders and Stroke (NINCDS). NCR demonstrates that many organizations working together can be more effective than single organizations working alone. Collective efforts in fiscal year 1985 appropriations achieved an 18 percent increase in funds for NINCDS, the largest increase for a single institute within the National Institutes of Health.

ASSOCIATION STRUCTURE

Legislative Council and Executive Board

ASHA members establish policies for the association through the election of members to the legislative council and to the executive board. ASHA members also establish policy by expressing their needs and concerns to their elected officers. According to Article IV of the ASHA bylaws,

> The Legislative Council is the legally responsible governing body of the Association. It establishes the policies of the Association and exercises all powers except those reserved to the Membership or assigned to the Executive Board by these Bylaws. The Legislative Council may delegate such powers as it may determine.

The legislative council is comprised of 150 members elected by ASHA members in each state (including the District of Columbia as a state). The size of each state delegation is proportionate to the number of ASHA members in each state as of 1978. Thus, the California and New York delegations are the largest, with each having nine councilors currently. The president and the past president of the National Student Speech Language Hearing Association serve as members of the legislative council with full rights and privileges. The ASHA president serves as chair of the legislative council, and other members of the executive board serve as *ex officio* council members without vote. The legislative council meets once a year in conjunction with the annual meeting of the association. The legislative council adopts a budget for the subsequent year and deliberates on numerous policy proposals that affect the profession, members of the association, and persons with communication disabilities.

Issues to be considered by each legislative council are published in abstract form in the October and November issues of the association's house organ *Asha,* along with the name and address of each legislative councilor. Members are encouraged to contact the councilors in their state about issues of concern to individual members. Sometimes the concerns expressed by one or two individual members can influence policies established for the association. For example, in the early 1980s the legislative council was considering proposed changes in the eligibility criteria for life membership. One member from North Carolina expressed concern about a specific criterion, and based on this one ASHA member's concern, the legislative council amended the eligibility requirements as originally proposed. A report of each legislative council meeting appears in the March issue of *Asha*, including the voting records of individual councilors.

Article IV, Section 2 of the ASHA bylaws states that

> The Executive Board is the legally responsible management body and shall supervise, control, and direct the affairs of the Association, and shall actively prosecute the objectives of the Association, operating in accordance with and administering and implementing the programs and policies established by these Bylaws and by the Legislative Council.

The executive board also monitors the activities of the national office through the executive director. The executive board consists of ten officers: The president, who serves as chair; the president-elect; the past president; the vice president for administration (who serves as treasurer); the vice president for clinical affairs; the vice president for education and scientific affairs; the vice president for planning; the vice president for professional and governmental affairs; the vice president for standards and ethics; and the executive director, who is nonvoting. The executive board meets three times a year (February, May, and August) to review proposed policy matters to be considered by the upcoming legislative council and to establish management directives for the association. In addition, the executive board meets annually for purposes of strategic, long-range planning.

Determination of policy by the legislative council and association management decisions by the executive board are guided by the bylaws of the association and the Strategic Long-Range Plan for the association adopted by the legislative council in 1983. In all events, ongoing activities must be consonant with the purposes of the organization as stated in its bylaws. ASHA legislative councilors and executive board members are not compensated for the services that they perform on a voluntary basis.

Activities of the association conducted to further ASHA's purposes are categorized into twenty-eight programs. These programs are as follows:

Minority
Research
Professional Practices
Foundation
Membership
Educational Standards Board

Professional Services Board
Continuing Education
Ethics
Clinical Certification
Student Affairs
Convention
Regional Conferences
Journal of Speech and Hearing Disorders (JSHD)
Journal of Speech and Hearing Research (JSHR)
Language, Speech and Hearing Services in Schools (LSHSS)
Asha
ASHA Directory
ASHA Monographs
ASHA Reports
Guide to Graduate Education
Guide to Professional Services
Special Reports/Brochures/Other Publications
DSHP
Public Information
Governmental Affairs
Retention and Recruitment
Governance

These programs are also used for presentation of the annual budget to the legislative council in that dollar expenditures are allocated to each of the programs. The statement of income and expenses also is categorized according to the designated programs.

Boards, Committees, and Task Forces

Most professional and trade organizations utilize a system of staff and voluntary member efforts to conduct the activities of the association. Some associations rely heavily on committees, with the staff providing primarily a support service (that is, vehicle for logistical coordination). Other associations rely heavily on staff to conduct the affairs of the association with monitoring by a board of directors and utilizing committees minimally. ASHA utilizes a system somewhere in the middle of the continuum. The affairs of the association are carried out by seven boards which have operational functions and by forty-seven standing committees which primarily study issues in a given area and provide recommendations to the executive board, and to the legislative council through the executive board. In addition, ad hoc committees and task forces are appointed when the need arises to study and make recommendation on a single issue. Staff persons are employed by the association not only to assist boards and committees in their activities but also to directly conduct certain activities for the association. Except for the Committee on Nominations, the Committee on Honors, and Committees of the Legislative Council, each standing committee (as well as each ad hoc committee and subcommittee) has a staff *ex officio* member who serves in a nonvoting capacity. Each task force is coordinated by a member of the staff, with a member of the executive board other than the executive director serving as liaison. All boards and committees of the executive board are monitored by a member of the board, generally one of the six vice presidents.

NATIONAL OFFICE

Staff activities are carried out within the association's headquarters building, known as the National Office. It is located at 10801 Rockville Pike, Rockville, Maryland, in proximity to the National Institutes of Health (NIH) and the Public Health Service. One block from a subway stop, the National Office is within a twenty- to thirty-minute ride from downtown Washington, the Capitol, and federal agencies such as the Department of Health and Human Services, the Department of Education, and the Department of Labor.

The operations of the National Office are under the direction of the executive director. Article IV, Section 3 b. states:

> Subject to the control of the Executive Board, the Executive Director is the chief administrative officer of the Association and in this capacity functions as Director of the National Office staff and operations, chief liaison and public information agent of the Association, contracting and financial officer of the Association, with authority to collect and disburse all funds of the Association, and business manager of the Association and its publications.

History of the National Office

In her book entitled *A History of the American Speech and Hearing Association 1925-1958*, Elaine Pagel Paden outlines the events that led to the establishment of the National Office. Until the National Office was established, the association's operations were handled by an officer of the association with considerable financial assistance from the officer's employing institution. For example, Dr. George A. Kopp, Wayne State University, served as secretary-treasurer from 1948 through 1956. Not only did Dr. Kopp supervise and conduct administration operations for the association, but Wayne State University also assumed the responsibility of providing a full-time administrative assistant. In 1953, the ASHA Committee on Association Planning noted that the association should not be dependent upon the subsidies (both in direct financial payments and in indirect contributions) from colleges and universities. A committee to study the establishment of the National Office was appointed in 1954. lengthy study was required before final decisions could be made on the city in which the National Office would be headquartered, the method of financial support, and the individual to fill the role of executive secretary.

The National Office of the American Speech and Hearing Association was officially opened on December 1, 1957, at 1001 Connecticut Avenue, N.W., Washington, D.C. Dr. Kenneth O. Johnson was selected as the first chief executive officer. Dr. Johnson was assisted by Luella B. Cannon, who currently serves as administrative assistant in the office of the executive director. In 1957, the annual budget for the association was $57,300.

Expansion of services for members and persons with communication disorders required an increase in staff and office space to handle the association's affairs. In 1964, a committee was appointed to project the association's facilities needs for the next ten years. A restricted housing fund was established, supported by a portion of each member's dues. (The housing fund exists today—of the $120.00 currently paid by members for dues and fees, $9.00 is allocated to the housing fund.) In addition to the housing fund, the then Office of Vocational Rehabilitation provided grants so that the association could construct and own its own headquarters building. These grants were procured through the efforts of Executive Secretary Johnson. A site was selected on Old Georgetown Road in Bethesda, Maryland, just off the NIH campus. The building was constructed for sole use by ASHA and was dedicated in 1966. At that time, the ASHA staff size was twenty-eight and its budget was $508,600.

The projections made by the committee in 1964 regarding the association's future space needs proved to be quite accurate. In the early 1970s, the association expanded its services to such a degree that the 16,000 square-foot-building on Old Georgetown Road was inadequate. (The existing building could not be expanded because of architectural and local government code reasons.) Rental office space was secured and the association embarked on an effort to acquire an appropriate site for a new headquarters building. In 1977, the association purchased a 30-acre tract of land and a turn-of-the-century mansion with approximately 19,000 square feet in space. The tract was procured with the understanding that the Corby Mansion would be used to house staff on an interim basis until new headquarters for the National Office could be constructed. At the time that the Corby tract was purchased, the staff size had grown to seventy and the association's annual budget had also increased, to $2,717,000.

The staff moved to the Corby Mansion in the summer of 1977. The association sold the mansion and surrounding eleven acres to Montgomery County, Maryland, in 1978 as the future home of the Strathmore Hall Arts Center; a lease-back agreement was secured from Montgomery County; construction of the new National Office was begun in 1979; and the current National Office Headquarters Building and Kenneth O. Johnson Education Center were dedicated in September 1981. At that time, the staff size had grown to eighty-six, and the budget increased to $5,092,000.

The current ASHA headquarters is located on an 7-acre tract, leaving an 11-acre parcel of land owned by the association for purposes of future development. The association currently is negotiating to develop the land as an association park to achieve two goals: (1) preserve the aesthetics of the property; and (2) generate steady revenue for the association in order to continue to carry out its programs.

National Office Organization

The National Office basically serves an administrative function; thus, the National Office is analogous to a business office. One necessity for the management of a business office is the establishment of a clear chain of authority. The chain of authority is the organizational structure of an office depicted by an organization chart. The ASHA National Office is organized into five departments in which there are divisions. In some departments, there are branches within divisions and sections within branches. The purpose of the organizational structure is to clearly demarcate who reports to whom; in other words, each employee has only one supervisor and is accountable to that supervisor for the fulfillment of job responsibilities. Each of the units has a director so that a section manager reports to a branch director, a branch director reports to a division director, a division director reports to a department director, and department directors report to the executive director. In turn, the executive director is accountable to the executive board. In addition, one office exists (the Office of Minority Concerns) whose director also reports directly to the executive director.

The current organizational structure was approved by the executive board in 1980 after considerable study and input from the executive board, members of the association outside the National Office, and expert consultants skilled in corporate/association organizational structure. The goal was to achieve an organizational structure that facilitated the administrative operations of the National Office in an efficient and effective manner. Few substantial changes have been made to the organizational structure since 1980.

Except for the Office of Minority Concerns and the administrative assistant in the office of the executive director, all staff members are related to one of the five departments. The *Administrative Department* is a support unit concerned with the conduct of the annual meeting and regional conferences, the management of information (that is, automation of association operations), and maintenance of the building's facilities.

The *Business Management Department* is responsible for the financial operations of the association that include record keeping for the approximately $8 million in accounts receivable and accounts payable, which involve thousands of business transactions annually. This department also is responsible for publications and marketing, which entails the printing production of the journals (except *Asha*), the *ASHA Directory, Guide to Graduate Education* and *Guide to Professional Services*. Marketing entails the procurement of advertisements in the journals as well as marketing other products of the association.

The staff of the *Governmental Affairs Department* focuses on federal and state laws and regulations that affect the profession, the practice of speech-language pathology and audiology, and individuals with speech, language, and hearing problems. Legislative concerns at the federal level focus on appropriations for programs that support research in human communication and its disorders, education and training of professionals, and delivery of services to individuals with communicative disorders. In addition, ASHA's activities with respect to federal legislation key into certain statutes such as the Education For All Handicapped Children's Act (P.L. 94-142), the Rehabilitation Act of 1973, as amended, the Medicare and Medicaid programs, and Maternal and Child Health Services. After laws are enacted by Congress, regulations are developed to implement these laws. Regulations are as critical as the legislative statutes themselves.

Unlike other organizations that have a single governmental focus, ASHA must key upon regulations that relate to a number of statutes concerned with education, health, and rehabilitation. Although most of the regulatory efforts are directed toward programs administered by the Department of Education and the Department of Health and Human Services, other federal departments are involved with aspects of our profession, such as the Department of Labor for the Hearing Conservation Program administered by the Occupational Safety and Health Administration, and the Department of Defense, which administers the CHAMPUS program for services to children of military personnel. The Governmental Affairs Department has intensified its efforts with respect to the federal third-party reimbursement programs (that is, Medicare and Medicaid), as well as to private sector health insurance programs. At the state level, efforts have been renewed to increase the number of state licensing laws as well as to study more intensively health insurance programs administered under state law. State regulatory efforts are directed primarily to state education departments' certification requirements.

The *Office of Minority Concerns* is responsible for the provision of programmatic and technical assistance to the executive director, members, association committees and other organizations and agencies relative to the service needs of the communicatively handicapped among racial/ethnic minority populations and the professional, research and training interests of racial/ethnic minority members. This office is a separate unit within the National Office organizational structure and cooperates with all departments within the National Office relative to minority concerns. The director of the Office of Minority Concerns functions under the direct authority of the executive director.

The *Professional Affairs Department* focuses its efforts on facilitating the needs of the research community within the association and the profession; procuring federal and private foundation grants and contracts (which allow the association to conduct special projects for its members and for the communicatively disordered); maintaining programs for membership recruitment and retention; processing applications for membership, certification, Educational Standards Board and Professional Services Board accreditation; facilitating efforts related to ethics, and continuing professional education; and providing technical assistance in speech-language pathology and audiology.

No matter how well constructed the organizational chart, the success of the inner workings of any office depends upon the ability of individuals to interrelate. Such ability is built on personal respect for individual talents and skills. Communication is also built on the premise that staff members are employed for one purpose: to foster the programs of the American Speech-Language-Hearing Association, the

American Speech-Language-Hearing Foundation, and the National Association for Hearing and Speech Action, in order to provide more and better services to members as well as to individuals with disorders of language, speech, and hearing.

The *Public Information Department* has two major foci. The most important of these is embodied in its name, whereby efforts are made to increase public awareness about disorders of human communication and services available to diagnose and remediate them. Specifically, this National Office department has developed public service announcements, arranged talk show placements, prepared news releases, and assisted in the development and placement of articles in popular magazines. These efforts are aimed at heightening general public awareness about (1) disorders of human communication; (2) the services that speech-language pathologists and audiologists provide; and (3) the fact that ASHA, as well as the National Association for Hearing and Speech Action, are appropriate contact resources. Annually, thousands of inquiries from the general public are received by the National Office, to all of which responses must be given. In addition to the general public, the Public Information Department seeks to enhance a level of knowledge about our profession among allied disciplines such as special educators; school administrative personnel (i.e., superintendents and principals in local school districts); and allied health professionals including physicians, psychologists, occupational therapists, physical therapists, nurses, and hospital/nursing home administrators. The department also provides programs designed to assist members of the association develop public information programs in their own local jurisdictions.

The second unit within the Public Information Department is concerned with editorial, graphics, and printing of many of the association's materials. Specifically, the unit is responsible for layout, design, production, and most of the writing of the journal, *Asha.* In addition, the graphics used on association, foundation, and NAHSA brochures, flyers, workbooks, posters and other informational materials are designed by staff persons.

National Office Accountability Systems

Duties of staff members within the National Office can generally be categorized as *operational* and *project.* Most positions contain both types of responsibilities, although project-oriented activities are more likely to dominate at the managerial levels than at the clerical levels. Word processing, bookkeeping, and membership/certification review all tend to be operational activities. Conduct of workshops, development of the budget, and application of computer programs are examples of efforts that are considered project oriented.

The first step in the association's accountability system is the development of a position description for each staff member. Some job descriptions are generic in that several staff members essentially have the same responsibility because the sheer volume of work cannot be accomplished by one individual. Generic job descriptions have two elements in common: (1) the responsibilities are the same (or essentially the same); and (2) the skills necessary to fulfill the responsibilities also are essentially the same. Other job descriptions are specific to the individual filling the position. The nature of the responsibilities changes from time to time with respect to the needs of the association; likewise, the qualifications and skills of the individuals filling the positions influence the outcomes for the responsibilities assigned.

Accountability for personnel is primarily achieved through the development of annual objectives above and beyond routine duties. Routine duties include answering telephone calls, responding to correspondence, completing forms as required, and other such day-to-day routine activities. In addition, most staff members (particularly those at more senior levels) develop a set of objectives annually, outlining what each staff member intends and is expected to accomplish during the calendar year. These objectives are not developed within a vacuum. Rather, staff members gather in meetings to go from a set of tentative activities to an officewide coordinated set of objectives to further the association's mission. Many of the activities have been recommended by boards or committees of the association; some activities are designed to facilitate certain endeavors in which boards and committees are engaged. Most National Office activities relate to the long-range plan for the association established by the legislative council in 1983.

Annually, the ASHA executive board reviews the proposed objectives. After the executive board has approved objectives for the forthcoming year(s), the staff member enters these objectives onto a project assignment record (PAR). Both the objective and the project assignment record are formatted in such a way that one can determine (1) what is to be done; (2) who is responsible for doing it; (3) to whom is it to be done; (4) when is it to be done; and (5) the criterion for success. The project assignment record further details the steps involved in order to accomplish the objective by the given date. In other words, the PAR represents a way of organizing the activities required to accomplish an objective in a sequential fashion in order to minimize potential problems. For example, the objective for one staff member might be the conduct of a workshop related to the development of accounting systems in speech-language and hearing clinics. The proposed overall plan and the date for the formulation of the proposed plan is cited on the PAR. The plan will include the proposed site, date, place, and description of the program. In greater detail, the plan will contain proposed content, proposed faculty, marketing plan, and budget. Based on the budget, the registration fee will be established. The PAR then states the steps by which approval of superiors is required, either separately or as part of the plan. A detailed series of action steps are outlined as to when informational/marketing brochures must be developed in-house, when they are to be sent to the printer, when they are to be returned by the printer, and when they are to be mailed to members.

Detailed planning (that is, PARs) is critical for achieving success in meeting objectives and for avoiding errors which can be costly to the association not only monetarily but also with respect to public relations. The consequences of error in many association projects conducted by staff are substantial. An error in dates on the brochure describing an upcoming conference not only results in extra effort in dollars to correct the mistake but creates a negative impression about the efficiency of the National Office. With the myriad activities conducted by the association to accomplish various projects to reach certain objectives and fulfill the long-range plan, some errors are bound to occur. However, ASHA's accountability system within the National Office is designed to minimize the occurrence of major errors—and, in some instances, to absolutely ensure against a catastrophic error occurring.

Salary Administration

ASHA allocates a substantial percentage of its financial resouces (about 45 percent) to personnel salaries and benefits. Thus, it is of interest to many members to know how staff salaries are determined.

ASHA currently uses the federal pay scale to compensate employees (except for the executive director and the few persons not housed in the National Office) in terms of a salary. Each position description is classified into one of eighteen grades by an independent personnel consultant. The consultant is selected by the association on the basis both of the number of years of experience he or she has had classifying jobs according to the federal pay scale, and on the basis of his or her updated knowledge about current trends in employee compensation. Within each grade, there are ten steps. For some positions, the first step within the grade is used to determine salary for a new employee. Other employees are hired at a given grade and/or step with an opportunity to advance a grade or advance step(s) after a certain period of employment with the association and after having demonstrated the ability to fulfill responsibilities of the position in a satisfactory manner. For other positions, the step within the grade is determined by such relevant factors as market supply and demand, or the particular skills of the individual taking the position. When individuals believe that their responsibilities have substantially changed over a period of time because of new responsibilities being added to their position or restructuring within the National Office, the staff member may request a reclassification review by the independent personnel consultant. An office review of all position descriptions is undertaken approximately every three to four years.

Salary increases occur in two ways: (1) step(s) within grade on the anniversary date of employment; and (2) adjustment of the federal pay scale by the president of the United States.

National Office Policies

Internal policies for the operation of the National Office are established by the executive board and/or the executive director with respect to officewide matters. The executive board approves those policies that have direct cost implications such as the establishment of the staff development program, modifications in the fringe benefits package, and the establishment of superior achievement and performance monetary awards program. The executive director determines those officewide policies that do not have substantial, direct budgetary implications such as the establishment of the flexitime program, job sharing, and expense reimbursement procedures. Unit directors often establish policies and procedures specific to the operations of that particular unit.

Prior to establishing or modifying office policies, staff input is sought when appropriate. Generally, input is obtained for those policies that will directly affect certain categories of employees or all employees. Staff input is received via suggestions placed in the "voice box" or during the process of the executive director's annual performance appraisal.

Major office policies are contained in the *Employee Personnel Handbook*. This handbook is given to all new employees, and an orientation session regarding the policies of the National Office is provided by the new employee's supervisor. Plans are currently underway to establish a more systematic orientation to new employees. In addition, *Staff Notes* is issued periodically. Because few policies can be established where there are no exceptions and cover all possible situations, *Staff Notes* serves to clarify and interpret existing policy as well as to remind staff members to adhere to current practices. *Staff Notes* also provides general information regarding ongoing activities within the National Office and the association.

Recruitment and Employment of National Office Staff

ASHA is an equal opportunity and affirmative action employer. Specific efforts are made to encourage applications from ethnic minority members, women, older persons, and disabled individuals. All positions are advertised internally to the National Office and many are advertised externally as well. By legislative council mandate, certain positions must be advertised to the ASHA membership. These positions are generally senior level positions, often with a preferred background in speech-language pathology, audiology, or speech and hearing science. Because of the association's policy to promote from within the organization, qualified applicants who are currently employees sometimes are given preference positions at a higher level than they currently hold.

When a position becomes vacant, a search team comprised of two to five staff employees is established. Résumés are reviewed in accord with predetermined, weighted criteria with respect to qualifications of applicants for the position. Applicants deemed to be the most appropriately qualified for the vacant position are scheduled for interviews. The number of interviewees is dependent upon the search team's determination regarding the qualifications of applicants.

When interviews are conducted, applicants are asked generic questions in addition to questions specific to themselves. In other words, if a particular qualification is deemed essential for the position, each applicant is asked about her or his strengths in the essential area of required expertise. Preferred qualifications are probed during the interview as deemed appropriate by the search team.

Following consensus of the search team after the interview, and with the approval of the direct line supervisor, an offer for employment is made to an individual. When the potential employee of choice has verbally agreed to accept the position, a written contract is drafted. The written contract is either the completion of a Notice of Employment form specifying salary and major fringe benefits, and/or a letter of agreement between the association and the employee. All contractual agreements for senior level positions are approved by the executive director.

Individuals who desire information about employment opportunities at the ASHA National Office can obtain such information by: (1) responding to notices that appear "At Press Time" and in the classified advertisements in the journal, *Asha*; (2) forward a brief résumé to the Personnel Branch to be kept on file for notification when employment opportunities become available; (3) respond to vacancy notices that are sent by mail to ASHA members; and/or (4) subscribe to the Employment Referral Service which lists not only position vacancies within the National Office but also position vacancies elsewhere.

CONCLUSION

It is the purpose of this chapter to provide the reader with an understanding of the total association structure, by means of which policies are formulated and actions taken. The reader will realize that the association is large and complex and that its members have a wide-ranging diversity of needs. As part of the structure set up to address these needs, a National Office with paid staff is maintained by the association. The executive director is in charge of the operations of the National Office, including the employment, promotion and termination of staff members. Vigorous efforts are made to increase the efficiency and productivity of National Office staff and its operations through systematic and defined procedures. The National Office operations are reviewed by a voluntary executive board, and the staff of the National Office strives to facilitate the work of ASHA members, boards and committees of the association, the executive board, and the legislative council.

12 Summary Comments

Herbert J. Oyer

The remarks that follow comment briefly upon some of the highlights of the preceding chapters. Each of the chapters has been written with current and future administrators in mind, and depending upon their focus, deal directly with the administrative process or present specific information of importance to the administrator; both in some instances.

There are a number of topics that are pertinent to the discussion of administration of speech-language-hearing units irrespective of their particular settings. Above all there is a matter of the administrative strategies that are employed in management. These vary from autocratic to highly democratic approaches wherein the policy making and implementation are the responsibilities of the faculty and/or staff. In contrast with most business and industrial operations, the personnel of speech-language-hearing units work collectively to formulate the objectives, implement the procedures to meet the objectives, and evaluate the outcomes. This is generally not difficult, for the employees of such units are professionals who work under the same code of ethics and share similar professional values.

Health insurance is a factor of vital importance to units delivering services to those sustaining communicative disorders. Recent data indicate that across the health field, approximately 29.5 percent of health costs are paid by private third-party sources; 28.06 percent from patients; and the remainder from federal, state or local public sources. A publication by the American Speech-Language-Hearing Association (Downey et al, 1984) on health insurance is extremely helpful to one responsible for administering clinical programs.

The profession has developed well, and makes an effort to protect society from untrained persons becoming involved in delivery of speech-language pathology and audiology services through national certification and state licensure of professionals. Likewise, the profession has set minimal standards for accreditation of both educational and service programs. Attention by administrators to these as well as other state and federal laws on nondiscrimination and the rights of the handicapped is imperative.

As for leadership, the point is made very clearly that effective communication is the vehicle of foremost importance for achieving consensus. Leaders are good listeners, trustworthy, and accessible. They believe in their cause and are sensitive to the need for development of staff personnel. It is fortunate if the administrator in charge of the speech, language and hearing unit is recognized as the leader.

The field of speech, language, and hearing is relatively young, particularly so in its profesional applications. As yet there is no agreed upon name to identify workers in the disorders of communication aspect of the field save for the terms *speech-language pathologist* and *audiologist*, which identify the professionally trained persons who render clinical services to those with communicative disorders. Throughout its development the field of communicative disorders has shown a continuing concern for standards and the quality of professional education and training, as well as for the service rendered to the public.

Although, as previously stated, there are common characteristics in the administration of speech, language and hearing programs irrespective of the particular setting, the differences among programs such as those operating within the hospital, public school or university immediately imply ground rules and responsibilities that are specific to each setting.

The university setting is unique because of the training of speech-language pathologists and audiologists. Not only must the administrator be concerned about the client and the clinician but also about the students as well. When clients come to the clinic they are interested in the finest service available, as is the administrator. It presents a particular challenge to communicate to clients that they will be interacting with students in training. As in any other setting the university program administrator is concerned with evaluation of performance both in the educational and training programs and in the service to the public. The accreditation programs of the American Speech-Language-Hearing Association provide the impetus for adhering to the minimal standards set by the profession.

The public school setting has, for the administrator, some of the same characteristics as those found in the university programs. Additionally, however, the clients seen are principally children, which implies interactions with teachers and parents. One of the most pervasive influences on programs for the communicatively handicapped in the public schools is P.L. 94-142. It has in a very direct way shaped the organization and administration of services. There is a mandate for more direct monitoring, supervision, and reporting by public school speech-language pathologists and audiologists than ever before. This has resulted in a greater accountability being required of those responsible for administering programs.

Programs that are community-based, because they must deal with professional staff and provide services to clients, place the same demands on the administrator as do programs in other settings. There are various models of organization for speech, language, and hearing programs that are described as community-based. Some are freestanding and report to a board of directors drawn from the community. Others have community governing boards but are nonetheless directly affiliated with educational and training institutions. Their administrators and staff have university appointments and are responsible for educating and training students who aspire to be speech-language pathologists or audiologists. In a way the administrator in this type of setting serves two masters: university and community. In this setting the matter of budget making and administration can be somewhat complex.

The program administered within the hospital is one that in more recent years has become more complicated because of the increasing complexity of the health care process. One of the distinguishing characteristics of the setting is that the speech, language and hearing patients are receiving services within a structure that is providing many other health services as well. Additionally, the speech-language pathologists and audiologists are surrounded by other health care personnel. Unless the hospital has teaching functions, it is somewhat different from the university-based clinical program. Because it is surrounded by other health professionals it is quite different from both the university and community-based programs unless the university program is one in which a medical school and/or rehabilitation program is a part of the scene. The speech, language, and hearing program administrator in the hospital setting reports, if the program is an autonomous department, to a vice president or perhaps directly to the president. In any case, the responsibilities of the administrator are highly similar to those in other settings as he or she deals with patients/clients and with the professional personnel who are responsible to them for provision of services.

Unlike civilian centers, the military speech, language and hearing programs are centrally administered and are guided by a basic military medical philosophy, the focus of which is to conserve fighting strength. Although administration is from a central source, the same knowledge and skills that are required of successful administrators in other settings are also required of the military administrator. Units for which the administrator is responsible are widely separated, which adds a unique factor. However, the administrative function is greatly facilitated through modern means of communication and transportation.

Although programs of speech, language, and hearing within the context of the Veteran's Administration are guided by decisions made at the central office, there are significant differences among programs. Speech, language and hearing as a service is independent and reports to the chief of staff of the VA. Likewise each local chief of speech and hearing service answers to the chief of staff of the particular medical center, and therefore conforms to the policies of the center. The administrator/chief is principally concerned with provision of quality care, participating in the training of medical care professionals, conducting research, and coordinating VA medical center care with care provided by community programs. Insofar as the human interactions with personnel are concerned, they are no different from those demanded of the administrator in other settings. Personnel selection follows guidelines that are set for all federal agencies. Likewise remuneration for professional services of staff members is a matter of federal pay schedules associated with government service (GS) levels. The similarity between VA and university programs is their common interest in training graduate students and the discovery of new knowledge through research.

Administration within agencies of government whose focus is that of research and training as well as supporting extramural research and training operate under a well-defined mission statement. Functions of branches of the agencies are also well-defined. Their personnel selection process is guided by the general criteria and rules set by government. Those responsible for such programs at any level have administrative demands made on them that call for many of the same skills as those required by one who directs, for example, the education and training of students within the university setting and the clinical program that helps to provide that training.

The National Office of the American Speech-Language-Hearing Association, insofar as its role and mission are concerned, is quite different from any of the direct education, training, research, and service-providing units of speech, language, and hearing in the various settings described. Here the policies and procedures are developed for guiding and monitoring the development and practice of the profession in this country. This is accomplished through a very orderly organizational format to include elected officers, councils, boards, committees, and task forces. The National Office is controlled by the executive board, composed of officers elected by the membership of ASHA. The administrator, who carries the title of executive director, manages a sizeable office force. This calls for the recruiting of personnel, and the evaluation of their effectiveness. Although it is a private enterprise, the federal pay scale is the model followed. Once again, even though the mission of this speech, language, and hearing enterprise is quite different from those in other settings, the principles of administration related to planning, budget, personnel management, program evaluation and general accountability are the same as for other units. The everchanging composition of the executive board and legislative council undoubtedly adds to the complexity of the administrative task.

The knowledge demanded by the administrators in the various settings and the process by which goals are attained vary substantially from setting to setting as do the constraints that are peculiar to particular types of settings. The general skills involved in communication, planning, allocating of responsibilities and deriving maximum output from staff are quite similar across settings.

REFERENCES

DOWNEY, MORGAN, STEVEN C. WHITE, AND SUSAN KARR. (1984). *Health insurance manual for speech-language pathologists and audiologists.* Rockville, Md.: American Speech-Language-Hearing Association.

Appendix I

Information contained in this chapter was obtained from a variety of Department of the Army regulations (AR), Department of the Army circulars, and Department of the Army pamphlets and training bulletins. The following list is a representative sample of the aforementioned information.

ARMY REGULATIONS

AR-10-6	Organizations and Functions: BRANCHES OF THE ARMY
AR-40-1	Medical Services: COMPOSITION, MISSION AND FUNCTIONS OF THE ARMY MEDICAL DEPARTMENT
AR-40-2	Medical Services: ARMY MEDICAL TREATMENT FACILITIES GENERAL ADMINISTRATION
AR-40-3	Medical Services: MEDICAL, DENTAL AND VETERINARY CARE: See Ch. 9 "Auditory Evaluation and Hearing Aids"
AR-40-4	Medical Services: ARMY MEDICAL DEPARTMENT FACILITIES/ACTIVITIES
AR-40-5	Medical Services: HEALTH AND ENVIRONMENT
AR-40-501	Medical Services: STANDARDS OF MEDICAL FITNESS
AR-40-66	Medical Services: MEDICAL RECORDS AND QUALITY ASSURANCE ADMINISTRATION
AR-611-101	COMMISSIONED OFFICER SPECIALTY CLASSIFICATION SYSTEM
AR-623-105	OFFICER EVALUATION REPORT SYSTEM

PAMPHLETS, CIRCULARS, BULLETINS, INSTRUCTIONS

DA PAMPHLETS 570–4	MANPOWER PROCEDURES HANDBOOK
DA PAMPHLETS 600–4	Army Medical Department: COMMISSIONED OFFICER PROFESSIONAL DEVELOPMENT AND UTILIZATION
DA CIRCULAR 600	Personnel Procurement: MEDICAL SERVICE CORPS AND VETERINARY CORPS ACTIVE DUTY PROGRAM BY FISCAL YEAR
TB MED 501	HEARING CONSERVATION
DoDI 6055.3	SUBJECT: HEARING CONSERVATION

Information about obtaining army regulations can be obtained from the Adjutant General Publications Center, 2800 Eastern Boulevard, Baltimore, Md. 21220.

Appendix II

Beneficiaries of hearing aids under the Program for the Handicapped, Office of Civilian Health and Medical Program of the Uniformed Services (CHAMPUS) must meet the following criteria:

1. Patients must be immediate dependents (spouse or children) of a service member.
2. Hearing examinations must be conducted by an audiologist, or supervised by an audiologist.
3. An otologic examination must be conducted by an otolaryngologist.
4. Speech recognition tests must be conducted at the patient's optimum hearing level (PB maximum).
5. Children may be tested by the best available measures of hearing evaluation (e.g., play, behavioral audiometry).
6. Hearing Impairment Criteria
   A. Testable patients
      1. Pure tone hearing loss
         Testable patients should be tested for pure tone hearing loss at 1,000, 2,000, and 3,000 Hz. Testing at 500 Hz should not be required as part of qualification criteria.
         a. Monaural hearing loss
            Patients should qualify for a hearing aid if testing shows a 45 db HL or poorer in either ear at either 1,000, 2,000, or 3,000 Hz frequencies.

   b. Binaural hearing loss
      Patients should qualify for a hearing aid if testing shows a 30 db
      HL or poorer in each ear at either 1,000, 2,000, or 3,000 Hz fre-
      quencies.

2. Speech discrimination handicap
   It might be possible for a patient not to meet the criteria for pure
   tone hearing loss and still be considered seriously handicapped because of severe speech discrimination impairment. It was agreed that
   most patients with 60 percent or poorer speech discrimination are
   functionally impaired and should be considered seriously handicapped.

   a. Severe speech discrimination impairment
      Speech discrimination of 60 percent or poorer is considered *severe*
      and should qualify a patient for a hearing aid whether or not the
      patient meets criteria for pure tone hearing loss.

   b. Moderate speech discrimination impairment
      Speech discrimination between 61 percent nd 80 pecent is con-
      sidered *moderate* and should be referred for professional review
      for a determination.

   c. Mild speech discrimination impairment
      Speech discrimination of 80 percent or better is considered *mild*
      and should not qualify a patient as seriously handicapped.

B. Nontestable patients

1. It is recommended that some "nontestable" beneficiaries should receive a hearing aid until reliable testing is available (e.g., patients with
bilateral aural atresia). Adequate testing may not be available or reliable until the patient reaches an older age.

2. All other "nontestable" patients should be reviewed individually to
determine their qualification for hearing aids. (This is expected to be
a very small percentage of candidates).

Appendix III
Code of Ethics of the American Speech-Language-Hearing Association - 1983

(Revised January 1, 1979)

PREAMBLE

The preservation of the highest standards of integrity and ethical principles is vital to the successful discharge of the professional responsibilities of all speech-language pathologists and audiologists. This Code of Ethics has been promulgated by the Association in an effort to stress the fundamental rules considered essential to this basic purpose. Any action that is in violation of the spirit and purpose of this Code shall be considered unethical. Failure to specify any particular responsibility or practice in this Code of Ethics should not be construed as denial of the existence of other responsibilities or practices.

The fundamental rules of ethical conduct are described in three categories: Principles of Ethics, Ethical Proscriptions, Matters of Professional Propriety.

1. Principles of ethics. Six Principles serve as a basis for the ethical evaluation of professional conduct and form the underlying moral basis for the Code of Ethics. Individuals[1] subscribing to this Code shall observe these principles as affirmative obligations under all conditions of professional activity.

2. Ethical proscriptions. Ethical Proscriptions are formal statements of prohibitions that are derived from the Principles of Ethics.

---

[1] "Individuals" refers to all Members of the American Speech-Language-Hearing Association and non-members who hold Certificate of Clinical Competence from this Association.

3. Matters of professional propriety.   Matters of Professional Propriety represent guidelines of conduct designed to promote the public interest and thereby better inform the public and particularly the persons in need of speech-language pathology and audiology services as to the availability and the rules regarding the delivery of those services.

PRINCIPLE OF ETHICS I

Individuals shall hold paramount the welfare of persons served professionally.

A. Individuals shall use every resource available, including referral to other specialists as needed, to provide the best service possible.
B. Individuals shall fully inform persons served of the nature and possible effects of the services.
C. Individuals shall fully inform subjects participating in research or teaching activities of the nature and possible effects of these activities.
D. Individuals' fees shall be commensurate with services rendered.
E. Individuals shall provide appropriate access to records of persons served professionally.
F. Individuals shall take all reasonable precautions to avoid injuring persons in the delivery of professional services.
G. Individuals shall evaluate services rendered to determine effectiveness.

Ethical Proscriptions

1. Individuals must not exploit persons in the delivery of professional services, including accepting persons for treatment when benefit cannot reasonably be expected or continuing treatment unnecessarily.
2. Individuals must not guarantee the results of any therapeutic procedures, directly or by implication. A reasonable statement of prognosis may be made, but caution must be exercised not to mislead persons served professionally to expect results that cannot be predicted from sound evidence.
3. Individuals must not use persons for teaching or research in a manner that constitutes invasion of privacy or fails to afford informed free choice to participate.
4. Individuals must not evaluate or treat speech, language or hearing disorders except in a professional relationship. They must not evaluate or treat solely by correspondence. This does not preclude follow-up correspondence with persons previously seen, nor providing them with general information of an educational nature.
5. Individuals must not reveal to unauthorized persons any professional or personal information obtained from the person served professionally, unless required by law or unless necessary to protect the welfare of the person or the community.
6. Individuals must not discriminate in the delivery of professional services on any basis that is unjustifiable or irrelevant to the need for and potential benefit from such services, such as race, sex, age, or religion.
7. Individuals must not charge for services not rendered.

PRINCIPLE OF ETHICS II

Individuals shall maintain high standards of professional competence.

A. Individuals engaging in clinical practice shall possess appropriate qualifications which are provided by the Association's program for certification of clinical competence.
B. Individuals shall continue their professional development throughout their careers.
C. Individuals shall identify competent, dependable referral sources for persons served professionally.
D. Individuals shall maintain adequate records of professional services rendered.

Ethical Proscriptions

1. Individuals must neither provide services nor supervision of services for which they have not been properly prepared, nor permit services to be provided by any of their staff who are not properly prepared.
2. Individuals must not provide clinical services by prescription of anyone who does not hold the Certificate of Clinical Competence.
3. Individuals must not delegate any service requiring the professional competence of a certified clinician to anyone unqualified.
4. Individuals must not offer clinical services by supportive personnel for whom they do not provide appropriate supervision and assume full responsibility.
5. Individuals must not require anyone under their supervision to engage in any practice that is a violation of the Code of Ethics.

PRINCIPLES OF ETHICS III

Individuals' statements to persons served professionally and to the public shall provide accurate information about the nature and management of communicative disorders, and about the profession and services rendered by its practitioners.

Ethical Proscriptions

1. Individuals must not misrepresent their training or competence.
2. Individuals' public statements providing information about professional services and products must not contain representations or claims that are false, deceptive or misleading.
3. Individuals must not use professional or commercial affiliations in any way that would mislead or limit services to persons served professionally.

Matters of Professional Propriety

1. Individuals should announce services in a manner consonant with highest professional standards in the community.

PRINCIPLE OF ETHICS IV

Individuals shall maintain objectivity in all matters concerning the welfare of persons served professionally.

A. Individuals who dispense products to persons served professionally shall observe the following standards:
   1. Products associated with professional practice must be dispensed to the person served as a part of a program of comprehensive habilitative care.
   2. Fees established for professional services must be independent of whether a product is dispensed.
   3. Persons served must be provided freedom of choice for the source of services and products.
   4. Price information about professional services rendered and products dispensed must be disclosed by providing to or posting for persons served a complete schedule of fees and charges in advance of rendering services, which schedule differentiates between fees for professional services and charges for products dispensed.
   5. Products dispensed to the person served must be evaluated to determine effectiveness.

Ethical Proscriptions

1. Individuals must not participate in activities that constitute a conflict of professional interest.

Matters of Professional Propriety

1. Individuals should not accept compensation for supervision or sponsorship from the clinician being supervised or sponsored.
2. Individuals should present products they have developed to their colleagues in a manner consonant with highest professional standards.

PRINCIPLE OF ETHICS V

Individuals shall honor their responsibilities to the public, their profession, and their relationships with colleagues and members of allied professions.

Matters of Professional Propriety

1. Individuals should seek to provide and expand services to persons with speech, language and hearing handicaps as well as to assist in establishing high professional standards for such programs.
2. Individuals should educate the public about speech, language and hearing processes, speech, language and hearing problems, and matters related to professional competence.

3. Individuals should strive to increase knowledge within the profession and share research with colleagues.
4. Individuals should establish harmonious relations with colleagues and members of other professions, and endeavor to inform members of related professions of services provided by speech-language pathologists and audiologists, as well as seek information from them.
5. Individuals should assign credit to those who have contributed to a publication in proportion to their contribution.

PRINCIPLE OF ETHICS VI

Individuals shall uphold the dignity of the profession and freely accept the profession's self-imposed standards.

A. Individuals shall inform the Ethical Practice Board of violations of this Code of Ethics.
B. Individuals shall cooperate fully with the Ethical Practice Board inquiries into matters of professional conduct related to this Code of Ethics.

Index

A

Academic training:
  and competency requirements, 80
  federal grant programs, 176, 178
  history, 21-23, 24-26
  hospital positions, 118-19
  management and marketing, 99, 116
  military programs, 142-43, 144, 146
  public school positions, 80
  student selection, 38
Accountability, 110, 199-200
Accreditation, 9, 22-24, 26, 27, 38, 205
  hospital programs, 102-3
  military programs, 141, 151
  university clinics, 48-49
Accreditation Manual for Hospitals
      (1985), 102, 107-8, 112
Adair, M. N., 77
Administration:
  of ASHA National Office, 195-203,
      207
  authority, chains of command, 1-3, 4
  community clinics, 84-99, 205
  hospital programs, 100-127, 206

  leadership, 30-35, 205
  and managerial training, 99, 116
  military programs, 129-55, 206
  public schools, 58-72, 205-6
  research programs, 174-89, 207
  universities:
    clinics, 41-51, 52, 205
    faculty and students, 37-41
  Veterans' Administration programs,
      161-64, 169-73, 206-7
Administration on Aging, 7-8
Advertising, 97, 126
Advisory committees, 96
Affirmative action programs, 7, 9
Aged clientele, 91, 101-2, 178
Age discrimination, 7-8
Air flow testing, 27
Allied health services, 112
American Academy of Private Practice
      in Speech Pathology and
      Audiology, 27-28
American Boards of Examiners in
      Speech Pathology and Audiology,
      22
American Dental Association, 22

American Hospital Association, 101
American Medical Association, 18, 22, 112
American Speech Correction Association, 25
American Speech-Language-Hearing Association (ASHA), 118, 119, 190-203
  accreditation, certification, licensure, 9-10, 22, 23-24, 112
  founding of (1925), 190
  membership, budget, staff, 190
  National Office, 195-203, 207
    accountability systems, 199-201
    address, 195
    history, 21-22, 195-96
    organization, 197-99
    personnel recruitment, 202-3
    policy making, 200, 201-2
    salary administration, 201
  nonprofit tax status, 190-91
  organizational structure, 192-95
    boards, committees, task forces, 194-95
    executive board, 193, 195
    legislative council, 192-93
    programs, 193-94
  program evaluation services, 77
  publications, 21-22, 192-93, 194, 197, 199, 202
    Code of Ethics, 6, 212-16
    health insurance manual, 5-6, 204-5
    supervision recommendations, 50, 78-79, 80
    supportive personnel guidelines, 120
  and related professional organizations, 191-92
  and state associations, 191
  Strategic Long-Range Plan, 193
American Speech-Language-Hearing Foundation (ASHF), 191, 199
Amplification systems, 91 (*see also* Hearing aids)
Ancillary services, 112, 176
Anderman, Bernard, 159
Anderson, Jean L., 49
Animal subjects, in research, 179, 185
Ansberry, Merle, 158-59
Aphasia, 15, 26, 119, 123
  federal grant programs, 177
  VA programs, 158, 168
Argyris, Chris, 3

Army Audiology and Speech Center (AASC), 138, 140, 144
Army Medical Department (AMEDD), 134-35
Army programs (*see* Military programs; Veterans' Administration)
Asha (journal), 21-22, 192-93, 194, 199, 203
ASHA Directory, 194, 197
Audiology:
  academic training, 119
  certification and licensure, 9-10, 26
  in community clinics, 91
  equipment and facilities, 17-18, 27, 107, 108-9
  fees for services, 117
  historical background, 14-18
  hospital programs, 101, 104, 106-10, 117, 118
  military programs, 131-55
  and otolaryngologists, 91, 139
  student performance evaluations, 50
  testing instruments, 27
  VA programs, 159, 160, 165, 168
Audiometers, 17-18
Auditory processing disorders, 26
Auditory training, 14, 18-19
Authority, line vs. staff, 58-59
Average response computers, 27

B

Balance, disturbances of, 177
Balich, S., 111
Barnard, C. I., 30-31, 34
Barnes, K. J., 76
Barry, Thomas J., 2
Beck, D., 113
Bekesy audiometry, 27
Bell, Alexander Graham, 15, 16, 18
Belt pneumographs, 15
Benefits, employee, 115-16
Berger, Kenneth W., 18
Berlin School for Speech and Voice Therapy, 15
Berry, Gordon, 130
Bess, F. H., 85
Bezold, F., 14
Bill Wilkerson Hearing and Speech Center (Nashville), 27, 85-92, 95-97

Bioacoustics Division (BAD), of Army
    Environmental Hygiene Agency,
    138, 141, 142, 144
Black, John W., 17
Blanchard, Kenneth, 4
Blanchet (French audiologist), 14
Blanton, Smiley, 17
Boards of education, 59, 61
Boston Stammerers Institute, 17
Bouchart, M., 110
Braidwood, Thomas, 14
Brainstem evoked response testing
    (BSER), 27, 109, 112, 118, 119,
    139
Brauckmann (Swiss lipreading teacher),
    19
Brazier, Mary A. B., 27
Broca, Paul, 15
Brown, D. G., 31
Bruhn, Martha, 19
Budgets (*see* Financial management)
Budoff, Milton, 7
Bunger, Anna, 19
Bureau of Education for the
    Handicapped, 21
Business office systems, 93-94, 99

C

Canfield, Norton, 131, 158
Cannon, Luella B., 196
Carhart, Raymond, 17, 23
Carhart notch, 27
Cerebral palsy, 86
Certificate of Clinical Competence
    (CCC), 9-10, 76, 117
  male vs. female holders, 154
  requirements, 10
Certification, 9-10, 23-24, 205
  hospital programs, 102-3
  military programs, 151-52
  public school programs, 75, 76-77, 80
  and signatures on forms, records, 111
Charge structures (*see* Fees for service)
Charvin (French physician), 15
Chemers, M. M., 31
Child Services Review System (CSRS),
    76
Chomsky, Noam, 26
Cineradiographic testing, 27

Civilian Health and Medical Program of
    the Uniformed Services
    (CHAMPUS), 153, 198, 210-11
Civil Rights Act of 1964, 8, 9
Civil rights movement, 56
Clark (computer scientist), 27
Clark, D. L., 58, 61
Cleft-palate disorders, 27
Cleveland Hearing and Speech Center,
    27
Clinical Fellowship Years, 76, 80, 106,
    117, 118
Clinics:
  accreditation, 9, 22, 48-49
  directors, 39, 51, 87
  history, 17, 22-23, 26, 27 (*see also*
    Community clinics; Military
    programs; Public schools;
    University clinics; Veterans'
    Administration)
Cluff, Gordon L., 23
Coen, R., 15
Community clinics, 84-99, 206
  business office systems, 93-94, 99
  diagnostic and therapeutic services, 86
  fees, 87, 89, 90
  financial management, 89, 90, 93-96
  hearing aids, 86, 91
  organization, 87-89
  outreach programs, 86-87
  patient composition, 86
  performance appraisal systems, 93
  planning, 93
  program development, marketing,
    96-97
  public and customer relations, 95, 96,
    97-98
  public school services, 8, 87
Computer technology, 51, 87, 173
Confidentiality, 10, 182, 213
Consultants, 95-96, 126-27
Coordinators, 62, 87, 89
Copyrights, patents, 10
Council on Accreditation of
    Occupational Hearing
    Conservation (CAOHC), 141, 152
Council on Accreditation of
    Rehabilitation Facilities, 103
Crawford, William L., 8
Crippled children's services, 98
Culatta, Richard, 49
Currier (U.S. audiologist), 18

Customer relations, 97-98 (*see also* public relations)

D

Data collection, 94, 109-10, 125, 141 142
Davis, P., 27
Day care programs, 97, 102
Deafness (*see* Hearing disorders)
Deleau (French audiologist), 14
del'Epee (French audiologist), 14
Department of Defense, 140-41, 198
Department of Education, 198
Department of Health and Human Services, 175, 184, 195, 198
Department of Labor, 198
Deschamps, C., 14
Developmental disabilities, 102
Diagnosis related categories (DRCs), 125
Dieffenbach, Johann F., 15, 16
Dietary services, in hospitals, 124
Dowling, Susann, 49
Downey, Morgan, 5, 102, 205
Drucker, P., 97, 100
Due process procedures, 7, 56
Dysarthria, 177
Dysphagia, 86, 123, 124

E

Earmold systems, 48, 108, 109, 139, 149, 161, 166
Ear trumpets, 14
Educational Standards Board (ASHA), 9, 22, 37, 38, 143, 198
Education of All Handicapped Children Act (P.L. 94-142), 8, 24, 198, 205-6
  general requirements, 71
  impact of, 56-57, 70
  part B amendments, 56
  speech-language-hearing requirements 71
  and state governments, 70
Eisenson, J., 26
Electronystagmography (ENG), 27, 109, 118, 119, 139, 149, 166
Elementary and Secondary Education Act of 1965, 21

Employee Personnel Handbook (ASHA), 202
Endicott, J., 133
Equal Opportunity Act of 1972, 9
Equal opportunity laws, 6-7, 9, 37, 56
Equipment:
  for audiology clinics, 17-18, 27, 107, 108-9
  for hospital programs, 107-8, 113-14
  for military programs, 150-51
  for university programs, 39
Ernaud (French audiologist), 14
Estes, Carroll L., 8
Ethics, 6
  ASHA Code, 6, 212-16
  and research subjects, 184-85
Europe, 13-15, 16, 19, 154
Evans, N. D., 59
Executive Order 11246, 7
Experimental Phonetics (Rousselet), 15
Expert witness testimony, 10

F

Fairbanks, Grant, 23
Family practice physicians, 113, 121
Federal Advisory Committee Act, 180
Federal agencies, funding, 20-21, 24, 98, 198
  and community clinics, 89-90, 94-95
  research programs, 175, 207
  and training programs, 24
Fees for service:
  in community clinics, 87, 89, 90
  in hospital programs, 116-17
  in university clinics, 43-44, 47-48, 52
Fein, D., 154
Feldman, A. S., 28, 90
Fiedler, F. E., 31
Financial management:
  of community clinics, 89, 90, 93-96
  of federal grants, 182, 187-89
  of hospital programs, 109-10, 113-17, 125-26
  of military programs, 150, 155
  of public school programs, 75
  of university facilities:
    clinics, 44, 46-48
    departments, 36, 38-39, 47
  of VA programs, 170

First Independent Research Support and Transition (FIRST) Award, 175
Fiscal years, 75, 170, 175
Flo Brown Memorial Laboratory (Wichita), 17
Flower, Richard M., 21
Fort Sam Houston (Tex.), 144, 146
Fourteenth Amendment, 7
Fowler, Edmund, 17
France, 13, 14, 15
Frank, Tom, 50
Freedom of Information Act, 179
Freeman, G. G., 73
French, T., 15
Froeschels (Austrian physician), 17
Fund raising, 95-96, 99

G

Gallaudet College (Washington, D.C.), 27
Galton-Edelman whistle, 14
Galvanic skin testing, 27
Garcia, M., 15
Gatza, J., 93
Germany, 13-14, 15
GI Bill program, 20, 161
Gifts, contributions, 95-96
Glorig, Aram, 158
Goble, F., 31
Goldberg, Steven S., 8
Goldstein (U.S. audiologist), 18
Governmental Affairs Department (ASHA), 197-98
Graduate interns:
  and clinical supervision, 43, 49, 50-51, 87, 118, 205
  in hospital programs, 106, 117, 118, 120-21
Grants, 94-95, 174, 175, 178-89
Great Britain, 13, 14, 15
Griffin, K. N., 77
Griffith, J., 102, 127
Group treatment procedures, 116-17
Gutzman, Albert, 15
Gutzman, H. Sr., 15

H

Haimann, T., 105
Halstead, W., 26

Handicapped children, 8, 56-57, 98
  (*see also* Education for All Handicapped Children Act)
Hardy, W., 26
Hartmann, A., 14
Healey, W. C., 76
Health Care Financing Administration (HCFA), 102
Health insurance, 24, 48, 98
  ASHA Manual on, 5-6, 204-5
  for professional staffs, 115
Health maintenance organizations, 98
Health Service Command (U.S. Army), 135-38
Hearing aids, 71
  community clinic programs, 86, 91
  electroacoustic characteristics, 160
  fitting fees, 48
  history of development, 18-20, 27
  hospital programs, 108-9, 117, 118
  military programs, 131, 139, 149, 153, 210-11
  VA programs, 151, 155, 159-61, 165
Hearing conservation programs, 87, 108
  federal programs, 198
  military programs, 133, 138, 139, 140-42, 152
Hearing disorders:
  federal grant programs, 177
  history of management, 13-14, 16
  incidence, in public schools, 54
  military programs, 130-31
  VA screening programs, 167-68
Hearing Evaluation Automated Data Registry System (HEARS), 142
Heinicke, S., 14
Helmholtz, Hermann von, 15
Helmick, Joseph, 49
Herzberg, Frederick, 3
History of the American Speech and Hearing Association, A (Paden), 195
Home health services, 86, 102
Hospital programs, 100-27
  accreditation, certification, licensure, 102-3
  administrative organization, 103-13
  authority, lines of, 103
  data collection, 109-10
  department identity, 104
  equipment, materials, 107-8
  facilities and space, 107
  patient scheduling, 105-6

Hospital programs (*cont.*)
  policies and procedures, 105
  quality of care, 109
  records and documentation, 110-11
  referrals, 112
  supervision of staff, 106
  financial management, 109-10, 113-17
  marketing, 126-27
  military facilities, 130, 136, 137,
    138 (*see also* Veterans'
    Administration)
  personnel management, 117-21
  services, 101-2, 112-13, 121-26
  wage and salary scales, 115
Housekeeping services, in hospitals, 125
Hughes, D. E., 14
Hughson, Walter, 131
Hunt (British stuttering expert), 15
Hutchinson (British physician), 15
Hutchinson, M. R., 18

I

Impedance testing, 27
Individualized Education Programs
    (IEPs), 8, 71
Industrial noise programs, 87, 108
Institutional Review Board (IRB), 185
Insurance programs, 115 (*see also*
    Health insurance, Medicare,
    Medicaid)
Intermediate school districts, 65, 73
Internal medicine, 113, 121
International Association of Logopedics
    and Phniatrics (IALP), 191
Itard, J.-M.-G., 14

J

Jacobson, L., 14
Jena method, of speech reading, 19
Jensen, T. J., 58, 61
Jerger typology, for Bekesy tracings, 27
Job descriptions, 105, 115, 199-200
Johns Hopkins University, 20
Johnson, Kenneth O., 22, 159, 196
Johnson, President Lyndon B., 21
Johnson, Spencer, 4
Joint Commission of Accreditation of
    Hospitals (JCAH), 102, 112, 152
Jones (U.S. audiologist), 18

Jones, Clarence J., 8
Jones, S., 76
*Journal of Speech and Hearing
    Disorders*, 17, 194

K

Karr, S., 102
Kastein, S., 26
Keys, John W., 46
Kindall, A. F., 93
Kinzie, Cora and Rose, 19
Knudson (U.S. audiologist), 18
Kopp, George A., 195
Kranz (U.S. audiologist), 18

L

Language disorders, 26-27
Larynx:
  diseases of the, 177
  observation techniques, 15
Laws, legislation, 6-9
  ASHA Government Affairs Dept.,
    197-98
  certification, licensure, 23-24
  training programs, 21 (*see also*
    Education of All Handicapped
    Children Act)
Leadership, 30-35, 81, 205
Learning disabilities, 26
Leigh Method, 16
Licensed practical nurses (LPNs), 122
Licensure, 9, 10, 23-24, 205
  of hospital programs, 102-3
  of military programs, 151
Likert, Rensis, 3, 5, 31
Line authority, 58
Lip and jaw movement testing, 27
Lipreading, 19-20, 130, 131
Livingston, J. S., 93
Loavenbruck, A., 109
Lobbying, 10, 56, 190
Long-term care facilities, 101-2

M

McGregor, Douglas, 2-3
Madell, J., 109
Maico Company, 18, 19

Malpractice, 10
Mama Lere Home (Nashville), 86
Management:
  of military programs, 139-42
  program evaluation procedures, 76-77
  theories, 2-5, 204
  training in, 99, 116
Marketing, 97
  ASHA publications, 197
  consultants in, 126-27
  hospital programs, 104, 116, 126-27
Martin Institute for Speech Correction
    (Ithaca, N.Y.), 17
Maslow, A. H., 31
Maternal and Child Health Services, 198
Medical directors, of clinics, 87
Medical records, 110-11, 125
Medical services, staff:
  in hospital programs, 112, 113,
    121-23
  in military programs, 131, 132, 133,
    134-35
Medicare, Medicaid, 5, 6, 24, 102,
    191, 198
Ménière's disease, 177
mental retardation, 26
Military hospitals, 18-19, 43 (*see also*
    Veterans' Administration)
Military programs (audiology), 129-55
  accreditation, certification, licensure,
    141, 151-52
  clinics, diagnostic and treatment,
    137-38, 139, 140, 151
  equipment, 150-51
  financial, budgetary issues, 150, 155
  hearing conservation programs, 133,
    138, 139, 140-42, 152
  history, 130-33
  management, 139-42
  medical philosophy, 134, 206
  organization, 135-38
  patient categories, 152-54
  personnel procurement, 142-48, 154
  staffing requirements, 148-49
  supervision, 139-40
Moehlman, A. B., 55, 57
Monochords, 14
Monthly operating reports (MORs),
    for hospital programs, 110
Morale, 41, 119
Morgenstern, Louise M., 19
Morrisett, L., 130, 131
Mueller-Walle, J., 19

Muller, J., 15
Muma, John R., 23
Myklebust, H., 26

N

National Advisory Neurological and
    Communicative Disorders and
    Stroke Council, 178, 185-86
National Associations for Hearing and
    Speech Action (NAHSH), 191,
    199
National Bureau of Standards, 160, 161
National Committee for Research in
    Neurological and Communicative
    Disorders (NCR), 192
National Council of Graduate Programs
    in Communicative Disorders and
    Sciences, 25-26, 36
National Council on Accreditation, 22
National Hospital for Speech Disorders
    (N.Y.C.), 17
National Institute of Dental Research,
    21
National Institutes of Health, 174, 175,
    179, 181, 184, 192, 195
National Institute of Neurological and
    Communicative Disorders and
    Stroke (NINCDS), 21, 174-89,
    192
  academic training, 176, 178
  applications, how to submit, 178-79
  Extramural Activities Program,
    176-77, 186, 189
  fiscal management of grants, 187-89
  program areas, 176-78
  research areas, 175-76
  review process, 179-87
    budget reductions, 182
    deferrals, 183-84
    initial review, 179-81
    priority ratings, percentile rankings,
      183
    project site visits, 181-82, 184
    secondary reviews, 185-86
    special consideration mechanism,
      186-87
  staff assistance, 189
  training activities, 176
National Research Service Award
    fellowships, 179

National Society for the Study and
Correction of Speech Disorders,
17
National Student Speech-Language-
Hearing Association, 192
Neagley, R. L., 59
Neurology, neurologists, 91, 104, 113,
118, 119, 122, 123, 167, 174, 177
News media, and program marketing, 97
Nitchie, Edward, 19
Noise-induced hearing loss, 87, 108,
133, 141
Northern, Jerry L., 133
Nursing homes, 101-2, 127
Nursing services, 101-2, 122-23

O

Occupational Safety and Health Act, 7
Occupational Safety and Health
Administration, 198
Occupational therapy, 40, 112, 123-24,
154
Oertel, M. J., 15
Office for Protection from Research
Risks (NIH), 184, 185
Office of Minority Concerns (ASHA),
197, 198
Ohio State University, 17
Older Americans Act of 1965, 7-8
O'Neill, J. M., 25
One-Minute Manager system, 4
Orenstein, Alan, 7
Orthopedic surgeons, 122
Otitis media, 54, 177
Otolaryngologists, otolaryngology,
104, 122
audiological services, 91, 139
in military programs, 130-33, 139
Otosclerosis, 27, 177
Outreach programs, 86-87, 118, 127

P

Paden, Elaine P., 25, 195
Patient-Care Audit System (PCAs),
76-77
Patients:
in community clinics, 86
in hospital programs, 105-6, 116,
117-18, 119
in university clinics, 39-40, 49-50
in VA clinics, 152, 159, 160, 166-68

Pediatrics, pediatricians, 113, 122, 123,
154
Percentile rankings, of research
applications, 183
Personnel:
ASHA National Office, 199-203
community clinics, 93
hospital programs, 106-7, 117-21
education, inservice and continuing,
109
job descriptions, 105
performance evaluations, 106-7
work schedules, 107
military programs, 142-48
audiology offices, 142-43
civilians in, 143, 147
officer professional development,
143-47
promotion systems, 147-48
public school programs, 74-75
universities:
academic departments, 37, 39-40
clinics, 42-43, 45-46
Veterans' Administration, 163-65,
169-70
Peterson, Gordon E., 23
Phonetics, experimental, 15
Physiatrists, 122
Physical medicine, 104
Physical therapy, 40, 112, 123, 154
Physicians:
as medical directors of clinics, 87
in military programs, 158-59, 162,
163
referrals from, 112, 167
and rehabilitation services, 113
specialists, 113, 121-22
in VA programs, 162, 163, 167
Pines, P. L., 76
Planning, Development, Management,
Evaluation system (PDME), 76
Pneumotachography, 27
Podemski, R. S., 56, 58, 64, 75
Politzer, A., 14
Porch, B., 26
Pregnancy Discrimination Act, 9
Presbycusis, 142, 167, 177
Principals, of public schools, 62-63
Privacy Act of 1974, 179, 182
Private practice, 27-28
Problem-Oriented Medical Record
(POMR), 110, 111
Productivity reports, 94, 114

Professional Affairs Department (ASHA), 198
Professional Services Board (ASHA), 9, 22, 48, 77, 103, 152, 198
Program development, 96-97, 193-94, 205 (*see also* Marketing)
Program planning and budget systems (PPBS), 75
Project assignment records (PARs), 200-201
Prospective payment system (PPS), 125
Psychiatrists, 122
Psychological services, 124, 154
P.T.A. groups, 61
Public Information Department (ASHA), 199
Public Law 94-142 (*see* Education for All Handicapped Children Act)
Public relations, 95, 96, 97-98, 99, 125, 199
Public schools, 24, 54-81
  administration, general, 58-63, 77, 205-6
    boards of education, 61
    directors, coordinators, supervisors, 62
    principals, 62-63
    superintendants of schools, 61-62
  community relations, 8, 57, 59, 61, 87
  incidence of speech and hearing problems, 54
  speech-language-hearing programs, 63-71
    administrative tasks, 74-79
    competency requirements, 79-81
    and handicapped children's act requirements, 70-71
    history of services, 16-17, 26
    organizational model, 66-70
    school districts, 73
    service commitments, 66
    service provision, 64-65, 74-75
    and state departments of education consultants, 72
    supervisory aspects, 77-79

Q

Quirk, John P., 7

R

Rabold, Ted F., 8
Racial minorities, 6-7, 9, 197, 198
Radiologists, 122
Rees, Norma S., 25
Referrals, 40, 123
  to hospital services, 112
  to VA programs, 139, 162-63, 165, 167, 168
Registered nurses (RNs), 122
Rehabilitation Act of 1973, 198
Rehabilitation services:
  in community clinics, 86, 98
  in hospital programs, 102-3, 112-13, 122-23
  in military programs, 130-31, 132
Research programs, 40-41, 87
  and ASHA assistance, 198
  ASHA projects, 191
  clinic laboratories, 39, 42, 43
  federal grant programs, 174-89, 207
  legislative concerns, 197-98
  military programs, 138
Research subjects:
  animal, 179, 185
  human, 10, 179, 184-85
Resource manuals, 74, 103
Respiratory care specialists, 125
Respite care facilities, 102
Rinne test, for hearing, 14
Rockey, Denise, 13, 15
Rosen, J., 98
Rotary accounts, in university clinics, 47
Rousselet, K., 15
Rowland, H., 103, 115
Rural areas, service provision in, 65, 126

S

Saxe, R. W., 58, 59
Schiefulbusch, R., 26
School districts, 58-61, 64-65, 73, 80
School planning, evaluation, and communication system (SPECS), 75
Schuell, H., 26
Secretaries, clerical staffs, 120
Sensory disorders, 177
Service courses, university, 40
Sex discrimination laws, 8-9

Shane, H., 110
Sheltered care facilities, 102, 127
Shrybman, James A., 7
Sicard Abbé R. A. C., 14
Signature form, on charts and records, 111
Silverman, Franklin H., 9, 10
Simon, Clarence T., 16, 22
Small Business Innovation Research Grants, 175-76
Smell, disorders of, 177
Smith College, 17
Social Security Act, 24
Social workers, 124, 154
Source Book of Health Insurance (1982-83), 5
Spahr, Frederick T., 6, 10
Special education courses, for public school program administrators, 80-81
Speech and Its Defects (Potter), 16
Speech-language pathology:
  academic autonomy of, 22-23
  certification and licensure, 9-10, 23-24, 205
  competency requirements for administrators, 80-81
  federal funding, programs, 20-21
  history, 15-17, 20-21, 130-31, 158
  military programs, exclusion from, 133
  national organization, growth of, 21-22 (*see also* American Speech-Language-Hearing Association)
  testing equipment, 27
  VA programs, 157-58, 163-73 (*see also* Audiology)
Speech Pathology (Travis), 17
Speech reading, 19-20
Spirometers, 15
Squires, Gregory D., 9
Staff authority, 58-59, 63
Staff Notes (ASHA), 202
State governments:
  certification requirements, 24
  community clinic liaisons, 98
  departments of education, 58, 72, 80
  handicapped children's services, 70, 71
  and public schools, 56, 58
State speech-language-hearing associations, 191
Stinchfield, Sara, 17

Strain gauges, 27
Strandberg, T., 101, 102
Stroke patients (*see* Aphasia)
Students, in university programs, 38, 44, 45, 48 (*see also* Graduate interns)
  grading, 51
  patient scheduling, 39-40, 49-50
  performance evaluation, 50-51
  supervisory duties, 42, 43
Stuttering, 15, 16, 17, 86, 177
Subjective, Objective, Assessment, and Plan system (SOAP), 110-11
Superintendents, of schools, 61-62
Supervisory tasks:
  ASHA list, 78-79
  in hospital programs, 106, 118
  in military programs, 139-40
  in public schools, 62, 77-79
  in university clinics, 43, 49-51, 52, 205-6
Swallowing disorders, 86, 123, 124
Switchboard operators, 125

T

Taste, disorders of, 177
Team approaches, 77-78, 176
Textbooks, 16, 17, 26-27
Thelwell, J., 15
Theories X, Y, Z, of management, 2-3, 4
Toynbee (British audiologist), 14-15
Training programs, 39
  and accreditation, 22, 24
  federal funding for, 20-21, 24
  federal grant programs, 175, 176, 179
  history of, 24-26
  in hospital services, 118-19, 120-21
  service courses, 40
  in universities, 24-26, 39, 40, 44, 205
Travis, L., 17
Truex, Edward H. Jr., 158
Tuning fork tests, 14

U

Universities:
  academic departments, 22-23, 36-37
  administrative responsibilities, 37-41
  curriculums, 38

faculty, 37-46
  clinic staff, 42-43, 45-46
  interprofessional relationships, 40
  meetings, 40
  morale, 41
  promotion, tenure, 37, 43, 52
  scheduling, 39-40
  suggestions to administrators, 51-52
  training programs, 24-26, 205 (*see
    also* Graduate interns)
University clinics, 41-51
  administrative models, 45, 205-6
  clinician-patient scheduling, 49-50
  community service agency links, 42
  directors' vs. chairpersons'
    responsibilities, 39, 51
  fees for service, 43-44, 47-48, 52
  financial management, 46-48
  patient scheduling, 49-50
  personnel management, 45-46
  professional staff, 42-43
  student performance, evaluation of,
    50-51
  supervision, 43, 49-51, 52, 205-6
  training programs, 39, 40, 44
University of Illinois, 24, 25
University of Iowa, 17, 20, 25
University of Michigan, 25
University of Wisconsin, 17, 24-25
Urbanschitsch, V., 14

V

Vanderbilt University School of
    Medicine, 85, 87
Van Hattum, R. J., 70, 72
Van Riper, Charles, 17
Vertigo, postural, 177
Veterans' Administration, 20-21, 27,
    133, 135, 157-73
  hospitals, 43-44, 101, 139, 165
  medical centers, 157, 158, 162-63,
    164, 169, 171-72
  organization, 157, 161-62
  speech pathology and audiology
    programs, 157-58, 163-73
    Central Office programs, 161
    decision making, 171
    financial management, 170
    hearing aid distribution program,
      151, 155, 159-61, 165

hearing screening programs, 167-68
history, 158-59
organization, 163-65
patients, 152, 159, 160, 166-68
personnel, 163-65, 169-70
professional relationships, 171-72
program management briefings,
    170-71
space criteria, 166
ten-year review program, 159
Videofluoroscopy, 123
Viet Nam War veterans, 8
Visiting Nurse Association, 102
Vocational Rehabilitation
    Administration, 21, 24

W

Walden, B., 133
Walter Reed Army Medical Center,
    130, 133, 136, 138, 140
Warren, Lillie, 19
Wayne State University, 195
Weber test, for hearing, 14
Weiss (Austrian physician), 17
Welsh, W. A., 31
Wepman, J., 26
Wernicke, Carl, 15
Wesley Wilkerson Society (Nashville),
    95, 96
West, Robert, 19-20
White, M. S., 102
White, Steven C., 102, 103, 112
White House conferences, 7, 17
Willis, W., 15
*Wisconsin Procedure for Appraisal of
    Clinical Competence*, 50
Women:
  in the audiology profession, 154
  and sex discrimination, 8-9
World War I, 130, 167
World War II, 20, 26, 130-31, 158, 159
Writing skills, 119
Written language disturbances, 124
Wyllie, J., 15

Z

Zero-based budgeting, 75